TOTAL HEALTH
THE CHINESE WAY

TOTAL HEALTH
THE CHINESE WAY

An Essential Guide to Easing Pain,
Reducing Stress, Treating Illness,
and Restoring the Body Through
Traditional Chinese Medicine

Esther Ting, PhD and
Marianne Jas, MA

Illustrations by Barbara Kolo

Da Capo
LIFE
LONG

A Member of the Perseus Books Group

Copyright © 2009 by Esther Ting and Marianne Jas
Illustrations copyright © 2009 by Barbara Kolo

Set in 10.75 point Warnock Pro

Library of Congress Cataloging-in-Publication Data

Ting, Esther.
  Total health the Chinese way : an essential guide to easing pain, reducing stress, treating illness and restoring the body through traditional Chinese medicine / by Esther Ting and Marianne Jas ; illustrations by Barbara Kolo. — 1st Da Capo Press ed.
       p. cm.
  Includes index.
  ISBN 978-1-60094-046-0 (alk. paper)
  1. Medicine, Chinese—Popular works. I. Jas, Marianne. II. Title.
  R601.T465 2009
  616'.09—dc22
                          2009024713

Published by Da Capo Press
A Member of the Perseus Books Group
www.dacapopress.com

Note: The information in this book is true and complete to the best of our knowledge. This book is intended only as an informative guide for those wishing to know more about health issues. In no way is this book intended to replace, countermand, or conflict with the advice given to you by your own physician. The ultimate decision concerning care should be made between you and your doctor. We strongly recommend you follow his or her advice. Information in this book is general and is offered with no guarantees on the part of the authors of Da Capo Press. The authors and publisher disclaim all liability in connection with the use of this book. The names and identifying details of people associated with events described in this book have been changed. Any similarity to actual persons is coincidental.

Da Capo Press books are available at special discounts for bulk purchases in the United States by corporations, institutions, and other organizations. For more information, please contact the Special Markets Department at the Perseus Books Group, 2300 Chestnut Street, Suite 200, Philadelphia, PA 19103, or call (800) 810-4145, ext. 5000, or e-mail special.markets@perseusbooks.com.

10 9 8 7 6 5 4 3 2

TO ALL OUR READERS:

May you have a life full of health, love, and longevity.

Contents

6

ADOPT A POSITIVE LIFESTYLE

How Your Habits Shape Your Health 151

7

MAXIMIZE YOUR ENERGY

Tuning In to Sun and Seasons 195

8

CLEAR OUT THE BLOCKAGES

Healing Techniques and Treatments 225

9

FOLLOWING NATURE'S PHASES

The Cycles of Life 263

Prologue

"Lie still, Marianne. Relax."

I barely felt the gentle push as the needle entered my toe.

"Good. Take a deep breath. Wonderful."

I nodded and steadied my breathing, eyes transfixed on a plastic statue of an odd little man perched on the bookcase. Naked and small in stature, he was covered head to toe in strange little red lines and black points. His lifeless eyes bored into me as the acupuncturist expertly maneuvered a row of needles up and down my body.

"Close your eyes. Let go." The doctor smiled. "I'll be back in a few minutes." She dimmed the lights and closed the door.

As the darkness settled over me, I asked myself once again, How did I get here? How did I end up so far from the doctors I had always trusted?

The whole thing began a few months earlier with a flu that felt like a lot of other flus. Fever. Lack of energy. Surely it would go away with some good nights' rest. But in a few short days the fever had given way to worse symptoms: acute exhaustion, dehydration, and vertigo. Suddenly, every bone was throbbing, every joint was on fire. My skin felt as if I had belly flopped on a barrel cactus. Some days I lived in a floating mist, unable to complete the simplest task; other days, I couldn't get out of bed at all.

My situation had gone from miserable to desperate. Never could I have imagined being this sick. The mere brush of fabric, the faintest tickle of bedsheet against my skin was excruciating. Driving was nearly impossible, and finally even eating became difficult. In a matter of weeks, the vibrant rosy-cheeked woman in the mirror had transformed into a chalky white shell. And as my body deteriorated, so did my mental state. How could this be? What horrible disease was attacking me?

The first doctor I visited recommended more rest; the second, a course of antibiotics. Both were pleasant, concerned, but neither treatment had any effect. A specialist even put me through a battery of blood and hormonal tests. Yet again, the results were inconclusive.

Beta-blockers were prescribed for the pain, but without saying so, my Western doctors were throwing up their hands. The closest anyone could come to a diagnosis was a condition known as chronic fatigue syndrome. As the months rolled by, it felt as if I had been abandoned by medical science, condemned to exist with this agony for the rest of my life. I resigned myself to being a prisoner in my own body, unable to live the way I always had.

Then, one day, a ray of hope appeared. While I was at my therapist's office, she mentioned Esther Ting, a Chinese doctor in Santa Monica who had successfully treated a number of her patients. This doctor, she told me, was getting positive results with chronic fatigue as well as other stubborn and often serious illnesses. My therapist had even taken her own daughter there—a teenager who had been diagnosed with an untreatable condition. The results had been nothing short of spectacular.

A Chinese doctor? I didn't exactly race to the phone. Wasn't this Chinese medicine the stuff of New Age disciples and aged hippies? As a former researcher, I believed in well-documented evidence supported by Western medical institutions. I found it fundamentally difficult to accept that a handful of needles and dried herbs could possibly heal an illness as serious as mine.

Ultimately, though, exhaustion and pain became the deciding factors. With nothing left to lose, the appointment was made. I *had* to try Chinese medicine.

The following morning I gathered my medical files and set out for this frontier of healing. The first signs were promising. Instead of battling for pricey parking atop a medical high-rise, I found myself in a leafy lot adjacent to a tidy office. Inside, the soothing tinkling of a tiny Chinese bell greeted me, my nostrils instantly seized by the earthy smell of herbs wafting through the waiting room.

A quiet, older Chinese man nodded hello, and handed me a few medical forms to fill out. He was Esther's longtime assistant and pharmacist. I would come to know Mr. Ma well.

After settling on the ornate yellow and red silk couch, I took a moment to savor the pots of bamboo, the fresh green tea and ready bowls of Chinese candies. Then, before I could even finish the forms, Esther herself burst out of an examination room. She wore a lab coat and smiled cheerily. "Come, come," she called, and waved me to a seat in her inner office.

Instead of holding forth behind an imposing desk, Esther clearly wanted to work up close and personal. Before I knew it, she was patting my hand, turning my palm upward and placing it on a wrist pad on her desk.

Esther began to work her fingers gently up and down my arm, starting from the wrist. Whatever she was doing, at least it wasn't painful.

I peered past her into the examining room. There didn't seem to be any of the usual devices to test heart rate or blood pressure. In fact, there was no equipment of any kind, just a small marble waterfall, trickling pleasantly in the background.

With both of my wrists in her hands, Esther looked deeply into my eyes and remarked on the redness of my cheeks. Then she opened my mouth. But instead of looking down my throat, she examined the tip of my tongue, commenting on the shape and the color. Okay. That's different.

As she continued to feel and listen, Esther peppered me with questions about my symptoms. How severe were they? How often had I experienced them?

Good. I was ready for this. Armed with X-rays and MRIs, blood panels and endocrine reports, I recited a litany of medical stats. Esther listened carefully, nodding all the while. Then she asked some odd questions:

What time of day did the nerve pains occur? Did I crave warmth? Was I more comfortable in the cold? Did I get thirsty a lot? How much food did I eat? Hot or cold?

I thought it was nice that she was so thorough, but wondered what any of this had to do with my condition. And how did she correctly determine I suffered painful menstrual periods, without even glancing at my charts?

After nearly ten minutes of these gentle palpitations and questions, Esther announced she was ready to discuss my diagnosis. Really? That quickly?

"Marianne," she began, "I am very confident I can heal your *physical* symptoms. It's not your extreme fatigue that troubles me. It is the stored accumulation of *emotions* I am reading in your body." Then she leaned closer. "Are you the oldest in your family? Because it's clear you have deeply held feelings of responsibility that have never been resolved and are affecting your liver."

Esther had only met me fifteen minutes ago. How did she figure out I was the oldest of three kids, and what on earth did my liver have to do with responsibility? And how was it possible she could get all that from reading my pulse?

I was about to respond when Esther patted my hand. "Marianne, listen to me. Up until now you have treated your body like an old car: When it got sick, you patched it together just to keep it on the road. But now the engine that keeps you going is broken, and the reason is simple. You have been holding onto anger and frustration for a very long time."

She explained that, over time, the corrosive effects of these emotions had attacked my body's organs and weakened their ability to function. This was made worse by accumulated stress as well as poor food and lifestyle choices.

"Your current symptoms are merely signals, Marianne. Your body has been talking to you but you haven't listened. Well, now it's time to overhaul that old car. Give me the gift of time and together we'll get the job done."

Over the following weeks and months, Esther and I worked closely together and my symptoms gradually eased. With every office visit I learned more about the causes of my crisis. She explained the vital role my liver played in balancing my body and why emotions are intimately connected to physical health. I learned the mechanics behind the "energy readings" that Esther performed along my arm and how they could reveal the inner health of organs and blood.

My illness wasn't just a random disorder; it was a warning signal. Somewhere along the way, I had let my emotional and physical reserves run down. I had become disconnected from my body. All of the "random" colds, flus, and infections that had dogged me from childhood were messages that I needed to change. Ignoring them meant there would be consequences when my immune system lost its ability to fight back.

Identifying a life-changing moment isn't always easy, but for me it happened while sitting in Esther's office staring at that naked statue. Somehow those crazy lines across the figure's plastic skin pointed to a journey I had to pursue. Tired of being sick, I handed myself over to an ancient healing tradition that to this day continues to amaze me with its power and effectiveness, even in the midst of the most modern medical discoveries.

I began my journey into Chinese medicine skeptical of its methods, wary that a three-thousand-year-old healing tradition could possibly have any relevance to my twenty-first-century life. But eight years later, after my own success story, and hearing the many stories of Esther's patients, I am a true believer.

Esther's lifelong dream is to bring Chinese medicine to the world, and I feel extremely fortunate to help her fulfill her purpose. In this book Esther and I want to introduce you to this ancient practice so that you may experience the same miraculous road to total health that we have. You will understand the root cause of most illnesses, and how they may be prevented using simple tools and techniques. And if you do get sick, you'll know exactly what to expect when visiting a Chinese physician.

So join us on this healing adventure. There's no better guide than Esther herself, and the ageless wisdom of traditional Chinese medicine.

Introduction:
A Doctor's Journey to Total Healing

This is a simple book. It's about health and healing. It's about the power of emotion. It's about preventing illness and how to get well.

After practicing Chinese medicine for over forty years, and nursing tens of thousands of patients back to health, I know one thing to be true: People *want* to be healthy, but they've forgotten how.

How can I be so sure? Because I've been there myself. I know what it feels like to have your body break down. And I have also experienced the incredible feeling that comes when the body heals from within, when energy returns and brings with it a new lease on life. For me, this journey began thirty years ago, when I almost lost my life.

In the fall of 1979, I had everything I could have hoped for. I was a popular doctor, with a thriving career at the local hospital in Shanghai. Although I loved my job, I was also devoted to my newborn son, Peter. It seemed as if life couldn't be more perfect—until that cool fall morning when I was jolted awake with pains so severe I could barely breathe. My lower abdomen was hemorrhaging badly, and within hours I found myself in my own hospital, helplessly immobile. I was losing vast amounts of blood, and the doctors needed to operate immediately. The diagnosis was dire: a large cyst in my fallopian tubes. Cancer.

As a physician and a descendent of a long line of Chinese doctors, I knew my life was in grave danger. Lying there in the darkness of my hospital room, trembling and weak, I thought about my family and young son, whom I adored and who depended on me. I still had such a bright future ahead, and so many things I wanted to accomplish.

Now *I* was the patient, and I had to make an important choice. Would I continue to fight? Or would I turn myself over to something greater and choose Western surgery?

By the time they wheeled me into the operating room, I had put myself in the surgeon's hands. I let go of my fear and my pain and surrendered to whatever fate had in store.

For the first time in a long while, I felt completely at peace.

The Path to Recovery

The news was good. My doctors pronounced the surgery successful, and after a course of both Western and Chinese treatments, I was soon recuperating at home. But the shock of my condition and my inability to read the signs continued to puzzle me.

I reread some of my old medical texts while reflecting on the work of my great-grandfather. His name was Ding Ganren, one of the most famous doctors in Chinese history, and personal physician to the last emperor of Shanghai. Known throughout China for his ability to read the human body, he was said to diagnose patients with infallible accuracy.

While staring at his picture, I found myself in a quandary. Even though I was clearly not yet as experienced as he, I had been working daily to perfect my diagnostic skills. Why had my own illness caught me so completely off guard? Why didn't I see the signs?

Suddenly, it was as if my great-grandfather, himself, was whispering in my ear: Your body *has* been sending you signs. You just

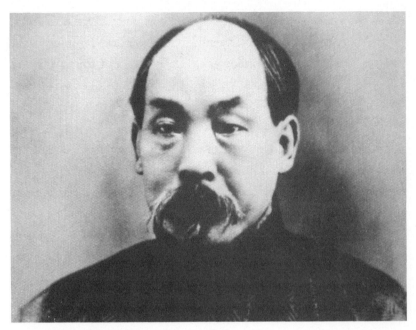

My great-grandfather, Ding Ganren

weren't listening. Your physical symptoms are just an outer manifestation of your emotions.

In an instant, I understood. Thousands of years ago, the ancient Chinese physicians discovered an important truth. When traumatic events happen, our body often traps those raw emotions in a *physical* form. By hiding and repressing unwanted feelings, we physically harm our body in the same way a toxic drug can slowly poison us.

I had been healing patients nearly every day for years, and yet all the while had been ignoring one of the most important principles of traditional Chinese medicine: the connection between health and *emotion.*

If I wanted to truly recover and follow in the footsteps of my family's honored medical tradition, I would have to learn to read my *own* body. I would have to look into my past and understand how it had affected my health. Only then could I truly heal my present and go on to discover my life's mission.

Clues from the Past

China in the 1940s and '50s was a turbulent time. World War II had just ended and a great famine was sweeping the country. I grew up as the oldest of five children, and my life was marked with a series of personal and family crises.

My parents, Dr. Ying Yu Wen and Dr. Ding Ji Hua, as well as my grandfather, Dr. Ding Zhongying, were all traditional Chinese practitioners, and ran a traditional medical clinic from our home on West Nanjing Street in the heart of Shanghai. Sadly, traditional Chinese practices were losing popularity in favor of Western medicine, and many clinics had closed.

In spite of having so many doctors in the family, I was a sickly child and contracted diphtheria. This was followed by a number of viral diseases and, eventually, tuberculosis. Using a combination of acupuncture and herbs, my family was able to cure me, but worse fortune was still to come.

At that time many doctors were called to practice medicine in far-flung provinces, and one day we got word that my father had been chosen. We were devastated, but there was no choice: he was obligated to go.

I'll never forget that gray November day in 1958, when I stood at the downtown station, watching my father board the train. I knew I would miss him terribly, and yet with four brothers and sisters to feed and a clinic still to run, we had to do what was necessary to survive.

My mother loved us very much but she had the clinic to run, so my sister and I took over the household. We cooked, cleaned, picked up herbal prescriptions, and did whatever was necessary.

A few years went by and traditional Chinese medicine slowly crept back into favor. In 1962, I was proud to be accepted into an elite medical program for the sons and daughters of well-known physicians, and there I began my own studies.

For my father, though, it was too late. He returned to us some years later in ill health, and died in my arms at the age of fifty from stomach cancer.

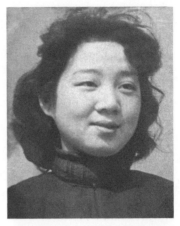

At eighteen years old, I contracted tuberculosis. My chubby cheeks are a result of the disease.

Burying the Past

Although we missed my father dearly, there was little time to mourn his passing. If I was going to become a doctor like my parents, I knew I had to bury my feelings and work hard.

In the following six years, I attended classes and studied late into the night, determined to do my best and continue my family's legacy.

My work at the hospital was exhilarating but exhausting. As luck would have it, I befriended a young man at the hospital pharmacy, who asked me to marry him. My parents approved of the match. As was customary at the time, I moved in with my husband's family, and soon afterward I gave birth to my dear son, Peter.

Now I was juggling career as well as the responsibilities of husband, son, and in-laws. And still I continued to bury the sadness and grief of my father's death. Somehow, though, I managed to keep it all under control—until that terrible fall morning, when I almost lost my life.

Lessons for Lasting Health

Looking back, my illness wasn't a mystery. The cancerous cyst was a physical manifestation of the underlying stresses that had built up

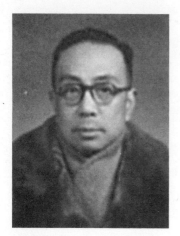

My father, Dr. Ding Ji Hua, at age forty-nine, shortly before his death

over the years. On the outside I was striving to be the best doctor possible, but on the inside I was masking a profound weakness. I had pushed myself beyond my limits, bottling up powerful feelings of anger, frustration, and sadness, until they expressed themselves in another way.

Three years later, I arrived in my new hometown of Santa Monica. Here, I found bright sunshine and ocean breezes. The mountains were nearby and I could walk to my office each day. This was the new beginning I had been searching for—the chance to finally take care of myself.

Each week I resolved to feel the sun's rays, to savor cool winds coming off the ocean, and to hike the mountain trails. I even created a daily exercise routine to move and strengthen my vital energy network and circuitry. Gradually, all of that pent-up grief began to dissolve. By releasing those heavy feelings, my body was finally taking the path to a strong and balanced Qi, or life force.

Now seventy-two years old, I have been cancer and illness free for thirty-five years. Despite a busy practice, I still feel healthy and full of energy.

What changed? My attitude. By altering the way I *thought* about my body, I transformed my life and my health.

The Three Principles

Today, my clinic in California treats patients with severe illnesses, some with conditions worse than mine had been. Like me, they want to know how it could have happened to them. They want to be healthy again and lead rich, productive lives.

Many times, when talking to new patients, I recognize the same telltale signs from all those years ago in China. Just as I did, they are working too hard, aren't getting enough sleep, and are burying feelings of frustration, sadness, and grief.

Many have already been treated by a long list of doctors, have spent a fortune on tests and medications, yet they're still sick and unhappy.

When I ask them to tell me about their body, they often look at me blankly. "I don't have *time* to pay attention to my body. Just fix me up. My children need me. My boss is relentless. I'm lucky if I make it through the day."

That's when I pass along three lessons I learned so many years ago. They're simple yet life changing, and after sharing them with tens of thousands of patients, I want to share them with you:

- **Listen to your body.** Your body is always trying to communicate. Don't ignore the warning signs.
- **Forgive and forget your past.** Live in the present. Holding on to the past is a major cause of illness.
- **Love your body.** Your body is a sacred gift. Treat it wisely and you will always experience the health and vitality that is your birthright.

What to Expect

In the chapters ahead, we will explore *why* you get sick and how to get better. We'll look at the human body and its intricate network of energy channels and power centers. We'll present simple, affordable healing foods, recipes, and herbs, and introduce invigorating new physical and mental exercises. We'll explore the powerful visualization tools and a host of meditative techniques and poses. You'll learn how to maximize your daily energy reserves, as well as discover helpful seasonal tips to create healthy, new lifestyle habits. And if you feel in need of professional expertise, we'll take you through the examination procedure of a Chinese doctor, so you'll know exactly what to expect.

Finally, you'll meet others who have made their own journeys to health. Sprinkled throughout are success stories drawn from over forty years of practice, including that of my coauthor, Marianne, who shares the journey of her own healing.

Total health has to do with the power you have over your fears and anxieties, and with your attitude toward getting well. So join me as we explore this gentle, ancient form of healing, and remember, it's *never* too late to enjoy the life you so richly deserve.

1

Understand How Your Body Works
Identifying Your Body's Power Centers

What does vibrant health mean to you? Running that marathon you've always wanted to enter? Picking up your child without excruciating back pain? Waking each morning rested and full of energy?

As a Chinese doctor I believe that the road to health doesn't begin with a pill or an X-ray, or even a visit to the doctor's office it begins with you. It begins with understanding your unique physical and character traits, the very essence of what makes you tick.

Chinese medicine is based on the principle that each person has a unique blueprint, an elaborate web of physical and emotional interactions and processes.

Your behavior, how you think, how you move—all are indicators of essential patterns and rhythms inside the body. These rhythms are sensitive and can easily become unbalanced long before any symptoms are visible on the outside.

To understand how Chinese medicine treats the body, it's necessary to use a whole new language. Western medicine tends to emphasize the specific purpose and function of each part of the human anatomy, whereas the Chinese physician looks at health as an inter-connected system, every element playing a part in the whole.

It's been said that the best way to understand the relationship be-tween these two healing traditions is by visualizing them as nothing more than different maps of the same surface. Each map shows the way to a healthier future, yet they approach the journey from paral-lel directions.

To see just how they differ set aside what you already know and journey back to the Han dynasty in China as it existed three thou-sand years ago.

The Five Power Centers

In ancient China, medicine was considered an art form. Many of the medical texts were written in a lyrical style, making them great mas-terworks of their time. Works included clever analogies and elaborate stories that went into great detail describing the human body. No wonder, thousands of years later, we find these metaphorical descrip-tions remarkably effective in helping us explain the role each organ plays.

Among these masterpieces is the *Nei Jing,* one of the world's first medical textbooks. Written in 200 BC, it looked at the body as a vast and mighty kingdom, complete with legions of guards to keep dis-ease at bay.

The master rulers of this body-kingdom consist of five major or-gans—the Liver, Heart, Spleen, Lung, and Kidney. These five pri-mary power centers, or *Zhang* organs, are supported by six secondary organs (or *Fu* organs). Each fulfills an important job within your body and each is connected in a unique way (see table 1-1).

The Masters: Zhang Organs

The leader or **king** of this internal realm is the **Heart,** and it has an essential function: to circulate Blood throughout your body in a steady, even flow. If your king is strong, your country will flourish. You are alert and aware. You are able to handle difficult situations and make wise decisions. A powerful Heart is fundamental to maintaining the rest of the kingdom in perfect harmony.

The **queen** of your kingdom is the **Lungs**. They support the Heart and govern the body's respiration. They also control your vital life force, or what we call *Qi* (pronounced chee). Think of Qi as the electricity that runs through your body. Qi is present in every living person, animal, plant, and organism in the universe. It is life's most basic energy force. When the Lungs are balanced and healthy, you breathe fully and deeply and your energy is strong. By bringing oxygen in, this organ enriches the Blood, ensuring that your energy reserves stay vibrant and healthy.

Next is the **commander** of your Blood, the **Liver**. This organ stores and governs the distribution of Blood throughout your body. It is the commander's job to tell the king how many of his troops (or Blood) should be deployed and where. When your commander is on the march, it's his job to make sure the Blood gets to its destination smoothly, and without a fight. A well-balanced Liver is considered a calm strategist who keeps the other organs in check.

The **ministry of power** is the **Kidneys**, which regulate energy and reproduction. Just as a country's electrical power is paramount to its survival, a healthy Kidney is the most important factor in your body's ability to function. For proper energy and drive, it has to work at peak efficiency.

The **ministry of food and agriculture** is the **Spleen**. As the organ in charge of your digestion, it watches over metabolism, transforming the food you eat into Blood and fuel. When balanced, it nourishes the cells and tissues critical for any healthy kingdom. Keeping the Spleen functioning well is absolutely essential for proper digestion.

The Royal Court: The Fu Organs

Your five primary rulers have complex responsibilities, and to succeed they need help. This is where the Fu organs come in. If not exactly leading members of the court, each of these organs supplies necessary services to make the kingdom function smoothly.

The Spleen relies on the **Stomach,** a close partner in the ministry of food and agriculture. The Stomach's job is to act as a food-processing center, receiving raw nutrients, assimilating them, and sending them on to the Small Intestine and Spleen.

TABLE 1-1. ORGANS AND THEIR RELATIONSHIPS

ORGAN	HEART	LUNG	LIVER	SPLEEN	KIDNEY
RELATED EMOTION	Joy Happiness	Sadness	Anger Frustration Stress	Worry Overthinking	Fear Anxiety Panic
RELATED EXTERNAL AREA	Complexion Tongue	Skin Nose	Nails Ligament Tendons Eyes	Mouth, Lips	Hair Bone Teeth Ears

The Heart's sister organ is the **Small Intestine**, your **food refinery**. This organ takes food from the Stomach and further refines, purifies, and redistributes it throughout the body. By enriching the Blood, it contributes to the strength of the Heart.

The Liver needs a wise and discerning **magistrate**, and that is your **Gall Bladder**. It is responsible for storing the bile from the Liver and sending it to the Small Intestine, where it's used for digestion. Your Gall Bladder also helps you to strategize, plan, and make sound decisions.

The Kidney's close partner is the **Bladder**. As **ministry of fluid management**, this organ's job is to assist the Kidneys in regulating and eliminating unnecessary fluids and toxins.

The Lung's faithful deputy is the **Colon,** or **Large Intestine.** This organ is considered the **ministry of waste management,** and is in charge of disposing the solid waste your body no longer needs. A healthy Colon cleanses and clears out unnecessary substances so that your kingdom can operate free of clutter.

In theory there is also a sixth Zhang organ: The Heart's protective guard, or **Pericardium**, which works closely with its Fu partner, the **Triple Heater**. This organ is responsible for your internal climate control: in charge of ruling the temperature of the upper, middle, and lower sections of your body. Both organs, however, are often considered part of the Heart's energy network.

Zhang and Fu: The Ultimate Power Centers

All of these organs are individual power centers. But they are also connected with one another by conduits called *energy channels*, the superhighways of energy that travel from one organ to the next. So when we refer to the Heart, Lungs, Liver, Spleen, or Kidneys, we're not only identifying the organ but also its accompanying circuitry. This is why throughout this book you will see Zhang and Fu organs capitalized, along with their companion energy channels and body fluids.

This hierarchy of leaders is a great way to visualize a complex series of internal actions. When your organs are healthy and supported by the court, your body can take in nutrients, then process and send them where needed. You make wise decisions and keep extreme emotions in check. But if you neglect the needs of your kingdom, upsetting the balance within, the walls of the castle will crumble, resulting in chaos, illness, and even death.

Your Five Power Centers: A Unique Role

Each of our power centers has a *physical* job—pumping Blood, digesting nutrients, distributing oxygen—but they also fulfill an even more important role, that of storing and managing your *emotions*.

This is where a Chinese physician comes in. By talking to my patients and carefully analyzing their signs and symptoms, I can uncover the cause of a complaint. It's usually right there, written in clues that are evident if one knows where to look. Unlike Western medicine, which considers the brain the central organ in charge of feelings, Chinese medicine teaches that human emotions reside in the organs themselves, and that the health of each organ can be read by external clues all over the body. For a Chinese doctor, the challenge is to read these clues, interpret them, and prescribe a treatment that will maintain a *balance* between your physical and emotional health.

To understand how the power centers perform their duties, let's look at each individually.

The Heart: Your Supreme Ruler

Think of the Heart as the supreme ruler of your body, the king of your castle. It is an energy system without peer. When it is strong, it pumps Blood throughout the arteries at a calm, peaceful pace. It also acts as a built-in climate control, regulating internal and external temperature and controlling your ability to sweat. If the Heart is working properly, it produces just the right amount of sweat to cool the body. But if the Heart energy network is weak, your temperature controls become unregulated, leading to dangerous conditions such as overheating and dehydration.

How can we tell whether the Heart is healthy or not? By reading specific signs on the *outside* of your body, a Chinese physician can determine a lot about the *inside* of your body (see figure 1-1). For example, a Western doctor might use a stethoscope to check your heart, whereas a Chinese doctor will observe your complexion, the sound of your voice, and the color and condition of your tongue (see chapter 8).

What the Heart Feels: Joy

Do you remember a time when you felt really happy? When you screamed with laughter at a classic comedy? Or when you fell so deeply and passionately in love you could barely contain yourself? Believe it or not, that's your Heart at work. In Chinese medicine, this organ signals the emotions of joy and love for another human being.

Having close and meaningful relationships is only possible when your Heart is in balance, when joy and passion are tempered with judgment. Wisdom also resides in your Heart and occupies a place called the *Shen*. This is the area that tells you when to be intimate and when to put distance between you and another person. It gives you the ability to make choices that are reasonable and sensible.

But when the Heart isn't circulating enough Blood, the Shen weakens and you lose that sense of personal boundary and space. Blood is pumped to the brain more slowly and judgment gets more

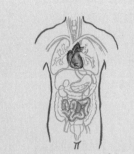

Figure 1-1. Symptoms of the Heart

**Signs of a Heart Network
in Balance**
Even pulse
Pink complexion
Balanced temperature
Strong circulation
Calm, even speech
Rational judgment
Even, happy temperament
Restful sleep

**Signs of a Heart Network
out of Balance**

*Symptoms of a **Weak** Heart Network*

Palpitations
Pale complexion
Low blood pressure
Night sweats
Shortness of breath
Chest pain
Lack of creativity
Low self-esteem
Tongue cracked along middle
Insomnia

*Symptoms of an **Overactive**
Heart Network*

Erratic pulse
Red complexion
Speech disturbances
Dark yellow urine
Blood in urine
Inappropriate laughter
Explosive energy
Hysteria
Insomnia

convoluted, causing mistakes and miscalculations. Emotional confusion follows, and it's easier to become nervous or, worse, lose perspective completely. There are examples of this everywhere, even in popular literature and movies.

This is why you should strive to keep your Heart at peace, pumping Blood regularly and rhythmically at all times. Living in a constant state of excitement or agitation only turns your mighty king into a flaming furnace, causing disturbed thought patterns, skin eruptions, restless sleep, and even swings in blood pressure.

THE HEART AND INSOMNIA

In Chinese medicine, the Heart houses the spirit, which includes thought processes, memory, emotions, and the ability to sleep. If you're having trouble dozing off, press the point between your eyebrows (Yintang) with your index fingers for approximately 30 seconds. A helpful herbal remedy, Tian Wan Bu Xin Dan (Celestial Emperor Pills) is often prescribed to help with this condition.

In coming chapters you'll learn some useful ways to avoid these perils as well as how to keep your Heart healthy, balanced, and strong.

Figure 1-1 presents many of the signs and symptoms associated with the Heart and its companion energy systems. A Chinese doctor will carefully consider each of these possible clues when evaluating your health.

The Spleen: Ruler of Nutrition

Together with its business partner, the Stomach, the pickle-shaped Spleen is considered the center of your body's digestive system. By absorbing the nutrients from your food and transforming them into Blood and Qi, the Spleen is the ultimate manufacturing and food processing plant. It not only fuels your ability to concentrate, it keeps blood vessels and muscles toned and healthy.

DIGESTION AND YOUR LIPS

If your lips are chronically cracked and dry, it can mean your Spleen has too much Heat and is not digesting properly, and you may not be producing enough Blood and Qi.

If your Spleen network is not functioning properly, it is impossible to assimilate the nutrients needed to give your body and mind the required amount of daily energy. Fatigue and exhaustion set in more readily, leading to digestive disturbances such as bloating, gas, and diarrhea.

The Spleen maintains the health of the muscles and also of the mouth. One of its jobs is to distribute Blood to this area, which means that the condition of the Spleen can be read by carefully observing the mouth. A healthy organ shows up with lips that are pink and moist, whereas a pale and cracked mouth with diminished saliva points to a Spleen that is underpowered.

What the Spleen Feels: Worry

With mounting credit card bills and looming deadlines, there's a pretty good chance you've been kept awake at night. The very act of worrying can cause imbalances that severely affect your health and well-being. Too much anxiety and overthinking affects your ability to think clearly and set goals. It's almost as if you can't digest your thoughts, and instead endlessly chew them over and over.

That's when the Spleen rebels. While you are in a constant state of anxiety, the spleen loses the ability to break down all of those essential nutrients you so badly need. It's a never-ending spiral. Expending so much energy on being anxious may cause you to lose the desire to eat, leading to such conditions as hypoglycemia, fatigue, and varicose veins.

The mouth is one area we can use to evaluate the Spleen and its companion energy systems, but a Chinese doctor also looks at other signs and symptoms when evaluating a health problem (see figure 1-2).

A Spleen Patient's Story: Geri

Geri was in the midst of a severe health crisis: nausea, vomiting, mental confusion, and painful muscle spasms in her left groin. And it wasn't anything new. For most of her adult life, Geri had suffered from a rare blood disease called porphyria, a deficiency in her blood enzymes. Every time she had her menstrual cycle these awful symptoms returned, and all she could do was curl up and wait for her painful period to end.

During my examination, I immediately saw that Geri was emaciated, her skin white, her lips pale and dry. This suggested that her Spleen wasn't able to do its job. As I spoke with her I gained a few more facts. Geri was five foot six, and weighed less than 110 pounds. She explained that no matter how much she ate, she never seemed to gain weight; this worried her so much she had lost the ability to focus or concentrate.

Without food, the body cannot create the Blood and Qi, the two primary Fluids vital to our body-kingdom that it needs to live, so my first job was to balance Geri's digestive organs. I targeted them with weekly acupuncture and herbs designed to jump-start her Spleen and Stomach. This allowed her to get the greatest benefit from her meals. Raw food could now be transformed into a nutritious soup that would form the foundation of her Blood and Qi.

Since Geri had been experiencing these symptoms off and on for the last thirty years, I cautioned that it would take a few months to fully nourish and strengthen her digestive organs. For her symptoms to disappear, her Blood and Qi needed time to build.

We started slowly, carefully adjusting the treatment to meet her body's response. I also prescribed protein soups as well as some easy massage techniques that would help Geri's digestive organs (see chapter 3).

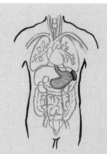

Figure 1-2. Symptoms of the Spleen

Signs of a Spleen Network in Balance
Healthy blood flow
Healthy blood sugar levels
Healthy digestion
Healthy weight
Good muscle tone
Strong focus, concentration

Signs of a Spleen Network out of Balance

*Symptoms of a **Weak** Spleen Network*

Slow healing of cuts
Bloating
Stomach pain
Low blood sugar
Yellow hands and feet
Dull headaches
Swollen, bleeding gums
Lack of saliva
Loose stools
Lack of appetite
Sugar cravings
Caffeine cravings
Poor muscle tone
Varicose veins
Exhaustion
Low self-esteem

*Symptoms of an **Overactive** Spleen Network*

Thick mucus in mouth, throat
Excess saliva
Water retention
Heartburn
Fluctuating blood sugar
Difficulty concentrating
Obesity
Excessive appetite
Swollen arms and legs
Weak joints, ankles, knees
Frequent bruising
Obsessive worrying
Overthinking/Pensiveness

After a few months of this treatment, she was feeling much better. She lost her severe menstrual symptoms and, as a nice benefit, had gained some fifteen pounds. Geri's case is a perfect illustration of how strongly two related power centers can hold influence over every aspect of your daily health.

The Lungs: Your Rhythmic Center

Like the Heart, the Lungs also have two important jobs. As your queen, they have the familiar job of breathing in oxygen, distributing it through your body, then expelling the carbon dioxide by-product. Then there is the other equally important task, managing the energy we call Qi.

WHAT IS QI?

Qi is life's most basic energy force and travels through the body by way of fourteen energy channels.

Qi exists everywhere, and is absorbed each time you take a breath. This "airborne" form of Qi is called *Da Qi*. The Lungs are in charge of processing this Qi and using it to fortify your Blood and energy channels. At the same time, the Lungs also exhale impure air and Qi with each outgoing breath, ensuring an even in-and-out exchange that keeps your body balanced.

This exchange of air is important so that Qi can flow smoothly from outside to inside and back again. Any disturbance in the Lungs' ability to maintain this exchange can result in a multitude of problems—chest pains, for instance, or possibly respiratory issues such as asthma or chronic bronchitis.

The two "gates," or openings, to the Lungs are the nose and the skin. If the organ is weak, the nose and sinuses are easily susceptible to outside viruses and infections. The skin is also considered the "Third Lung," so it can be the first line of defense when illness hits. To stay moist, the skin is dependent on the Lungs. That's why in Chinese medicine we say the skin's health reflects the health of our Lungs.

What can be done to determine whether the Lungs are carrying out their duties as they should? Unlike Western doctors, Chinese physicians don't use an MRI or an X-ray machine. Instead, we use an exam that pays particular attention to the exterior of the nose, the sinuses, and especially the skin (see figure 1-3).

What the Lungs Feel: Sadness

At some point in life it is inevitable that every person experiences loss. It might be the death of a loved one or an adored pet; even selling the cherished family home can feel overwhelmingly sad. Whatever the cause,

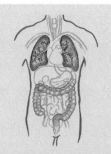

Figure 1-3. Symptoms of the Lungs

Signs of a Lung Network in Balance
Even, balanced breathing
High energy
Strong immune system
Strong circulation
Calm demeanor
Regular bowel movements

Signs of a Lung Network out of Balance

*Symptoms of a **Weak** Lung Network*

Tight chest
Breathing difficulties
Bronchial spasms
Cough
Dermatitis
Eczema
Pale complexion
Inappropriate sweating
Chest pain
Lack of inspiration
Trouble gaining weight
Sadness
Suspiciousness

*Symptoms of an **Overactive** Lung Network*

Shortness of breath
Acute sinus infections
Acute bronchial infections
Yellow or green mucus
Acute chest pain
Lack of perspiration
Dry skin, hair
Acute skin flare-ups
Acne
Other skin problems

the Lungs must manage and process these significant emotions of grief. At these times, it's easy for feelings of sadness and melancholy to become overwhelming, and if left unexpressed, they can lead to Lungs that are weak and unbalanced. This compromises the immune system, which in turn can make you excessively rigid and isolated.

The physical body will usually show symptoms of this. You might have difficulty breathing or experience constant bronchial infections. Some people suffer dry skin and dehydration, whereas others endure chronic acne and rosacea. These conditions are often brought on by long-repressed emotions of sadness, expressing themselves through the skin.

If you recognize these signs, it is very possible that your Lungs are holding on to deep residual feelings of grief.

Once again, by looking at figure 1-3, you can see signs and symptoms associated with the Lungs and their companion energy systems. For a Chinese doctor, all are important signals that determine the health of your queen.

MARIANNE JAS'S STORY: TAKING CARE OF MY QUEEN

It was a spring afternoon and I was in my first month of acupuncture treatment. My symptoms were clearing dramatically. I had renewed energy, and felt more alive and awake. Yet somehow my emotions had not caught up with my physical transformation. I still found myself encountering periods of depression and sadness.

The previous year had been a dark time emotionally: My husband and I had recently made some financially challenging career changes and had unexpectedly lost a beloved pet. For the first time in a decade, I was also feeling the deep disconnect between my West Coast life and that of my extended family in the east. Many people I cared about were far away and the separation wasn't anyone's fault but my own.

As Esther gently placed the needles on my arms and legs, she told me to breathe deeply, and that if I felt any emotions rise up, I should feel free to cry. I nodded politely and assured her that wouldn't be necessary. But she wasn't letting me off so easy.

"It's time for your queen to release all of this repressed sadness and recharge your energy channels," she said as she adjusted my pillow.

I remember letting the darkness settle over me and feebly trying to make sense of all this new jargon. The thought of my Lungs as queen, my Heart as king, my Liver as a general sounded more like a wild fairy tale than a credible medical treatment.

Like most people, I had had my health evaluated using numbers and measurements culled from expensive medical tests. My Lungs were defined in terms of units of capacity, my Heart by the rate at which it pumped. My Liver and Kidneys had specific BUN and creatine enzymes levels that demonstrated I was normal and healthy. So the idea of my body being an ancient kingdom, presided over by rulers keeping me healthy and strong, sounded pretty fantastic.

But that afternoon, in the warmth and comfort of Esther's darkened treatment room, I felt my resistance give way. Strong feelings from the past year welled up inside and I couldn't hold back. The tears began to flow, and, in a spontaneous flood my "queen" finally got the release she had been craving.

Afterward I fell into a deep thirty-minute sleep and, upon awakening, felt immensely relieved, as if a new energy was surging throughout my body. Could this be what Esther meant when she vowed to recharge my energy channels?

She certainly seemed satisfied. "Good, good!" she said as she removed the needles. "The Qi has shifted. Your kingdom has been at war for a long time, but now the conflict is ending and it's time to rebuild your body's leadership."

Esther promptly gave me the best homework assignment I'd ever had. Watch a comedy: film or TV show didn't matter. As she put it, "Laughter strengthens the whole Heart energy network, keeping your king healthy and strong."

It had taken me a while to reconcile the differences between Eastern and Western doctors, but after the successful results of my treatment got under way, the effectiveness of Chinese medicine was all too evident.

Once I understood the concept of our organs' having both a physical and emotional job, it was easier to imagine the magnificent kingdom within, its five rulers each with an important role to play. This notion became a vivid yet lyrical representation, and for me, one that has been immensely empowering.

The Kidneys: Your Body's Power Supply

The next time you feel tired or run-down, consider this: It may be your Kidneys talking. When working normally, they regulate the supply of water and fluids throughout the body, providing warmth, fuel, and energy to other vital organs, including the brain. As the body's water and power department, the Kidneys' job is to ensure the robust energy each of us relies upon to live.

It is water that makes it possible for waste products to be gathered and eliminated in the form of perspiration or urine. The Kidneys regulate this process, doing their part to ensure these fluids are properly transported and transformed.

Since the Kidneys' energy network extends all the way from your feet to your ears, they have a wide-ranging jurisdiction. Besides processing bodily fluids, these organs also regulate the health and growth of hair and hearing. In fact, everything to do with hard connective tissue in the body—bones, marrow, teeth—are part of the Kidneys' domain.

Even more significant, the Kidneys store your vital essence or what we call *Jing* (see chapter 6). From a Western perspective, Jing can be compared to a genetic code, a fundamental nucleus of information and energy that is given to each and every one of us at birth. As time progresses and your body grows older, you draw on this store, causing Jing to decline. This is why protecting the Kidneys is so vital to the aging process.

How does a Chinese practitioner know what's going on with your Kidneys? By examining the physical condition of your bones, teeth, ears, and hair: each a reliable indicator of your organs' health.

What the Kidneys Feel: Fear

When in balance, the Kidneys are your ultimate power players. Not only do they provide a major source of energy, they have a critical emotional job: to process past and present feelings of fear.

When your body is operating in an even, steady state, the emotion of fear can actually be beneficial. It alerts you to imminent danger and tells you when to fight or run. But when fear is a constant state of mind, your adrenaline never stops pumping; your blood vessels and muscles remain tight and contracted. Great if you're running from a polar bear. Not so good if you're driving carpool.

This is why it is so critical that the Kidneys stay well balanced. Living in constant fear or panic wears down the body's power department,

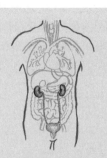

Figure 1-4. Symptoms of the Kidneys

Signs of a Kidney Network in Balance
Lots of energy
Confidence
Alert senses
Strong bones
Strong teeth
Thick, healthy hair
Acute hearing
Healthy urinary function
Healthy sexual drive
Creativity
Mental acuity

Signs of a Kidney Network out of Balance

*Symptoms of **Weak** Kidneys*

Low energy
Excessive fear
Pale skin
Low sex drive
Impotence
Infertility
Cold hands, cold feet
Prematurely gray hair
Blue-black circles under eyes
Hearing difficulties

*Symptoms of **Overactive** Kidneys*

Neurological disorders
Concentration issues
Gum disease
Urinary infections
Kidney stones
Lower back pain
Weak knee, hip joints
Premature ejaculation
Heightened sex drive

leading to symptoms that include depression, sore back and joints, problems with bones and teeth, as well as urinary and bladder dysfunction.

All of these signs, as well as those in figure 1-4, indicate Kidney dysfunction and can be evaluated to root out the primary cause of specific health conditions.

A Kidney Patient's Story: Mark

A female patient of mine called me, totally distraught. Her husband, Mark, had undergone a heart bypass operation some years before and his symptoms had suddenly returned.

Mark had been spending his nights in the emergency room for the past month, suffering from severe respiratory disruption and relying on oxygen to breathe. My patient was sure her beloved husband was dying and was frantic to know what could be wrong. Would I come over?

When I first saw Mark in his darkened living room, tethered to an oxygen mask, he was indeed a sorrowful sight. His legs had swollen to twice their normal size. He was so frail that he couldn't lift his head to greet me. His depression was so severe, he was getting little sleep.

I began by studying his face. He was pale, with deep blue-black circles under his eyes. When I took his hands, they were cold to the touch. It all added up. This time it wasn't his heart condition. The constant fear had compromised his Kidneys and upset the circulation of Qi through his body.

As I gently inserted acupuncture needles along Mark's Kidney points, I asked Mark when his symptoms had recurred, and soon discovered that they had coincided with a powerful earthquake that had hit the area recently.

This incident had severely traumatized Mark, and afterward he refused to sleep in his own house, for fear of aftershocks. His wife had finally coaxed him back inside, but Mark wasn't the same, convinced another quake meant certain death.

At this point, it was clear to me what had happened. I calmly told Mark what had happened to his power centers. The earthquake had produced a severe physical and emotional jolt to his system, and the fear had literally cut off his power supply. Because the Kidneys provide energy to all the other organs, there was a cascade effect. His Liver had lost the ability to control the volume of Blood, his Lungs had cut off the flow of Qi, and finally his Heart could no longer properly pump and circulate fluids.

The acupuncture treatments would help with the energy loss, but to jump-start his power centers he needed to get some sleep. I asked Mark to do some meditation as well as my internal organ exercises before bedtime and promised I'd be back the next day.

That night, he slept for the first time in months. The next evening, I rang the doorbell only to have it answered by Mark himself, who gave me a big hug. His swelling was gone and his breathing was normal. After only three days of treatment his symptoms had disappeared. It seemed incredible to his wife, but to me it was a perfect instance of how the body's vast power department can be shut down by something as simple as an uncontrollable emotion.

The Liver: Your Commander

Most of us know that the Liver cleans and prepares the Blood, but it has many other functions as well. It is the power center that arranges and sends out proper amounts of Blood and energy to all the cells in your body, a good explanation for why the Liver is sometimes called "the commander."

Among this organ's jobs, it is responsible for the even flow of Blood and Qi, and for keeping the body flexible. It makes sense, then, that the health of your tendons and ligaments relies on a Liver that flows in a strong smooth manner. If your commander can't send enough Blood to keep the tendons moist and supple, muscle spasms, tightness, and numbness in the limbs can follow.

BLOOD

Blood is considered the vital essence of the body. Blood is the mother of Qi, and is created by the Spleen from the foods that one eats. Part of the Blood's job is to moisten tissues and organs.

To get a good idea of what a Chinese doctor sees when diagnosing the signs and symptoms of an unbalanced Liver, take a look at figure 1-5.

Weak Liver function also can result in pale, brittle nails, another sign that something isn't right. Because the Liver's energy network extends the entire length of the body, it also supervises the health of the tendons as well as the functions of the eye. Not surprisingly, many eye diseases and disorders can be traced directly to the Liver.

What the Liver Feels: Anger

The physical job of cleansing and regulating the volume of Blood is one of the Liver's primary jobs, but equally important is its ability to keep your stress levels in check. By managing and processing strong emotions such as anger, frustration, and resentment, the Liver allows you to deal with life's bumps and set-backs. This makes it a key player in releasing excessive pressure and strain.

When the Liver is balanced, it sends out just the right amounts of Blood in an easy, relaxed rhythm. You feel calm and tranquil as you move through the day. But if these feelings are bottled up, that's when the Liver becomes irritable and cantankerous.

Repressing emotions can be a destructive habit. It creates a backlog, or what we call *Qi stagnation*. After a while, just about anything can make you furious: a fight with a parent, a late-night telemarketer, even a deep scratch on a new pair of shoes.

By holding rage inside your kingdom walls, you are weakening your commander, who is no longer able to tell his king when and where to pump Blood and Qi. Soon, all of this fury has free rein to rush through the body like a wind, creating a storm of symptoms: migraines, hot flashes, cramps, ulcers, PMS, even a heart attack or stroke. With time, Liver function becomes overworked, blocking the volume and flow of

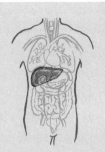

Figure 1-5. Symptoms of the Liver

Signs of a Liver Network in Balance
Even blood pressure
Even emotions
Calm demeanor
Strategic thinking
Rational decision making
Suppleness and flexibility
Strong eyesight
Healthy digestion
Regular menstrual cycle

Signs of a Liver Network out of Balance

*Symptoms of a **Weak** Liver Network*

Visual disturbances
Eye strain or spasms
Allergies
Bloating
Unstable blood pressure
Irregular menses
Infertility
Insomnia
Lack of energy
Depression
Substance abuse
Chest pain
Cramps

*Symptoms of an **Overactive** Liver Network*

Migraines
Severe eye strain
Cracked fingernails
Muscle spasms in head, neck
Tendon injuries
Sciatica
Heavy menstrual cycles
Acute chest pain
High blood pressure
Self-destructive tendencies

Blood. This leads to energy blockages and stagnation, a direct cause of painful conditions that affect both body and mind.

Anger, Qi Stagnation, and Chronic Disease

I was reminded of the importance of Liver function while on a vacation to stalactite caves in Pennsylvania. As I watched the water collect and drip from these calcified formations, I thought of them slowly forming over thousands of years. It occurred to me that the relationship between the body and serious disease is quite similar. Just as the stalactite accumulates size from the constant dripping, so can a tumor or cyst grow through stagnated cells caused by chronic anger and frustration. Eventually this constant "dripping" can lead to severe illness, such as cancer and heart attacks.

This is why we have to find a positive way to deal with these feelings; otherwise the Liver becomes a sponge, soaking up negative feelings and slowly compromising organ function.

Looking back, I am certain that the tumor I contracted at an early age had its roots in the repressed frustration and sadness of my own childhood. By allowing these emotions to fester, I was strangling the free flow of Qi and fluids, eventually inhibiting proper organ function.

When I consult with patients who are struggling with significant amounts of anger and stress, I urge them to find ways to release these emotions before they lead to something serious.

Releasing Emotion to Heal Ovarian Cysts: Susan

Susan hadn't even reached forty and yet her doctors had given her a terrible diagnosis: an inoperable ovarian cyst. She had been told that she would never be able to have a child, and that although her painful symptoms could be "managed," they would never completely disappear.

It was heartbreaking. Here was a person facing the same terrible diagnosis that I once had, and the first thing I needed to do was to put her at ease.

In the course of my career I have found that, in general, women tend to be more openly sensitive and emotional than my male patients. There are many benefits to this, of course, but there is one big disadvantage. When a person's energy channels become blocked by traumatic events—what I call "emotional garbage"—that person is sowing the seeds of illness. Clearly this garbage was at least partially responsible for Susan's condition.

As it turned out, I learned she had a trigger similar to my own—a tumultuous childhood. She had come from an abusive home, and although Susan felt she had come to terms with the ordeal, she had really only suppressed the trauma and accompanying anger. As the years went by, these strong emotions had taken a heavy toll on her body.

Traditional Chinese medicine considers an ovarian cyst a blockage that has lodged in the reproductive organs. Mostly, it's the result of Liver Qi Stagnation. In the case of a cyst, Liver Heat causes the Blood in the uterus to stagnate and block the Blood vessels, creating inflammation throughout the area.

Now I knew what I was treating. We began a course of acupuncture and herbs, and with Susan willing to unburden herself, we exposed many of her unresolved emotional issues. Eventually, the blockages eased, allowing Blood to once again circulate through her vessels. Surprising both Susan and her doctors, we eliminated the cyst, and her ovaries were pronounced healthy and ready to conceive a child.

Managing Your Emotions: Forgive and Forget the Past

Although explosive emotions are sometimes difficult to control, in an often complex world they are hard to escape. That makes channeling your emotions in a healthy manner all the more important. It's not always easy, but here's a good place to start. *Forgive and forget your past.* Recent studies are proving what Chinese medicine has known for centuries: that the act of forgiveness can have a radical impact on your health.

There is a growing field called psycho-neuroimmunology, an unwieldy word that simply means looking at how the brain and immune systems interact. This work is providing new insights and evidence into the connection between our innermost thoughts and their effect on our health.

Using new techniques, scientists now have a way to measure the connection between the brain and how the body experiences pain, pleasure, and other emotions. They have discovered evidence that the mere mental image of ease and forgiveness can produce positive endorphins that make *physical changes* in the body. Within the brain, these images are actually being accepted as authentic experiences.

When patients confide that some issue is making them angry and frustrated, I first ask them to put themselves in a restful state. Then, I have them imagine what their life would be like without the stressful issue. What new activities would they try? If they were free of the burden, what would their life look like instead? How would they feel physically?

You can use this same stress-relieving exercise to create a beneficial effect on your mind and body. By putting yourself in a restful state, you will allow your thoughts to open up and accept new possibilities. The ability to get a new job or fulfill a personal health goal can often be advanced by using this simple power of suggestion.

In addition, a variety of methods described in this book will also help. For instance, try rubbing the indentation between your big and second toe. Or use the meditation exercises described in chapter 5. Practiced individually or in combination, these tips will help to smooth the flow of Blood and Qi, benefiting not just the Liver but all of your organs.

By forgiving and letting go, you are giving your Liver the room to resume its job of continuing the smooth and even flow of blood, the very thing that opens your mind to new horizons.

FORGIVENESS AND YOUR HEALTH

A 2001 survey published in the *Journal of Adult Development* found that those people aged forty-five and older who forgave others had better mental and physical health than those who did not.

Understanding How Your Body Works

By understanding the basics of Chinese medicine, it's easier to appreciate the power that the Zhang Fu organs have over your health. You now know where they are located and what they are capable of. But this is only the first step in understanding your body. By mastering some simple tools and techniques you will learn so much more about why you get sick and how to avoid it.

Ahead, you'll discover how to care for yourself, especially for your immune system. You'll learn how to nourish your body with food and strengthen it with exercise so you can stop illness *before* it happens. And if you do get sick, you'll learn some basic steps to help you get well. My goal is to put you in the driver's seat so you can focus on healing fully and completely.

So, take charge of your health and change your life. If I did it, so can you.

OUR BODY KINGDOM

12 Major Zhang and Fu Organs. Inside all of us is a miraculous kingdom made up of five primary Zhang and five accompanying Fu organ systems. A sixth organ, called the **Pericardium**, and its partner the **Triple Heater**, are closely related to the Heart organ system.

5 Primary Zhang Organs

Heart: Pumps the Blood, related to the emotion of **joy,** rules the complexion and the tongue

- **Underpowered Heart:** Symptoms include palpitations, shortness of breath, lack of creativity.
- **Overactive Heart:** Symptoms include erratic pulse, speech disturbances, explosive energy.

Spleen: Regulates digestion, related to the emotion of **worry**, rules the mouth and the lips

- **Underpowered Spleen:** Symptoms include bloating, loose stools, lack of appetite, low self-esteem.
- **Overactive Spleen:** Symptoms include thick mucus, heartburn, frequent bruising, obsessive worrying.

Lungs: In charge of breathing and managing Qi, related to the emotion of **sadness**. Rules the skin and the nose.

- **Underpowered Lungs:** Symptoms include cough, eczema, lack of inspiration.
- **Overactive Lungs:** Symptoms include shortness of breath, dry skin and hair.

Kidney: Regulates the flow of water, related to the emotion of **fear**, rules the hair, bones, teeth, and ears.

- **Underpowered Kidney:** Symptoms include low energy, cold hands, feet, blue-black circles under eyes, fearfulness.
- **Overactive Kidney:** Symptoms include urinary infections, kidney stones, heightened sex drive.

Liver: Arranges and sends out the proper amounts of Blood, related to the emotion of **anger**. Rules the nails, ligaments, tendons, and eyes.

- **Underpowered Liver:** Symptoms include visual disturbances, irregular menses, cramps, infertility, depression.
- **Overactive Liver:** Symptoms include migraines, high blood pressure, self-destructive tendencies.

5 Fu Partners

- **Heart:** Small Intestine
- **Heart (Pericardium):** Triple Heater
- **Spleen:** Stomach
- **Lungs:** Colon
- **Kidney:** Bladder
- **Liver:** Gall Bladder

2

Strengthen Your Defenses
The Real Reasons We Get Sick

Many people come to me after everything else they've tried has failed. They've been to their family practice, they've been to their physician or neighborhood clinic, even the local pharmacist. They've spent thousands of dollars on tests and prescription medications, and still they don't seem to get better. No wonder the first question I'm usually asked is, "Why am I still sick?"

Western medicine has relies heavily on statistics and numbers. Blood pressure rates, endocrine levels, and EKG readouts often determine the difference between sickness and health. Of course, in many cases, these tests have proven immensely valuable, and certainly have saved lives.

But what if you fall through the cracks? What if the numbers point to perfect health but you still feel sick? A Western doctor might say the results are in the "normal" range, and there's nothing more he or she can do. The numbers may be accurate, but you know your body is in distress. What do you do then?

This is where Chinese medicine differs from Western. Rather than focusing solely on visible symptoms and test results, we look at the deeper *imbalances* inside and outside of the body. These imbalances are the key to uncovering exactly what is causing an illness or health condition

To understand how this works, consider Yin and Yang, the two sides in this critical balance.

Yin and Yang

Yin and Yang are intertwined yet opposite energies present within every human, animal, and living organism throughout the universe. Their interconnected relationship is displayed in the *Tajii*, a symbol many thousands of years old that unites both forces into one universal image (see figure 2-1).

The Yin energy, or black area, symbolizes a cool, calm state, while the Yang, or white area, is its active, fiery opposite. To maintain the best health, these reciprocal energies must coexist peacefully within the larger whole.

Try thinking of the entire human body as a reflection of these two forces. When people are healthy, they balance equal amounts of Yin and Yang. But when individuals lack this crucial equilibrium, it opens the door for foreign viruses, genetic diseases, and other conditions to establish a foothold.

Unfortunately, it's not hard for this to happen. Many people do it every day. They don't tend to their body's needs. They surrender to strong emotions and don't eat or exercise properly. They work too hard and weaken their defenses, making them susceptible to outside invaders. And when external forces beyond their control do cause an illness, they're not always aware of what their body needs to heal.

Once again, the body should be treated with an understanding of how its organs relate to one another. When Yin and Yang are balanced, your kingdom is prosperous; your coffers are filled with rich energy and nutrients. When your leaders are happy and content, they will rule with confidence, knowledge, and wisdom.

Your Kingdom's Defense System

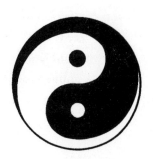

Figure 2-1. Tajii, the Yin and Yang Symbol

Throughout the ages, entire civilizations have stood or fallen depending on the strength of their defenses. Strong countries invade weak ones and kingdoms fall.

But the good news is that the human body has an impressive defensive guard—in China it is called the *Wei Qi*. In Western medicine it is known as the immune system.

A strong Wei Qi is the reason some people can go skinny-dipping in the ocean in the heart of winter without getting sick, whereas others get the sniffles the minute they get out the snow shovel.

To get an idea of what Wei Qi represents, let's go back to your imaginary kingdom. Visualize, if you will, thousands of troops spread out in formation as far as the eye can see, a massive force protecting your body-kingdom—your very own powerful Wei Qi army.

Like any army, these troops need a strong foundation. Feed them well, exercise them, keep their spirits up, and your Wei Qi will protect your body against hostile invaders. Remember, though, that an army needs to be supplied, and in the case of your body, those supplies consist of nutritious food, healthy air, water, and exercise. Even play and relaxation are important.

Four basic forms of Qi are essential to good health and a robust Wei Qi. The first is called *Original Qi*, or *Jing Qi*, the prenatal foundation of energy that you are born with. Second is *Gu Qi*, the energy you receive from the food you eat. Third is *Da Qi*, energy that comes from the air you breathe. Finally, there is *Shen Qi*, or the love energy you get from family, friends, and spiritual practice. If any or all of these forms of Qi become weak or fractured, your troops can't defend the kingdom and the door is left open to attack by illness.

How do you keep your army vibrant and powerful? Eat well, breathe deeply, love daily, and preserve the energy and the body you were born with.

This doesn't have to be hard, and it always begins with a strong Qi.

Ahead, we'll look at the many ways you can strengthen and preserve your Wei Qi and keep your immune system from a distressing fate. But first, let's investigate the circumstances and conditions that can lead to a breakdown. Like any strong kingdom, you need to know what and where the enemy is.

Why We Get Sick

When your Wei Qi, or immune system, is weakened, it's usually because one or more elements have been compromised. Maybe your energy troops aren't receiving rest or proper nutrition. Maybe they aren't getting exercise or are crippled by emotional distress. Any of these can lead to a weakening of your once mighty defenses, and, before you know it, illness follows.

Chinese medicine identifies four main sources of illness:

- **External causes:** viruses, bacteria, pathogens
- **Internal causes:** emotions, psychological trauma
- **Miscellaneous causes:** injuries, accidents
- **Lifestyle causes:** overwork, poor diet, social habits, inappropriate or lack of exercise

All these factors, by themselves or in combination, can have devastating effects on your health. To see how, let's take a deeper look at the first three categories.

The External Causes of Illness:
The Five Weather Devils

If you've ever left your winter jacket at home and had to walk head-long into an icy wind, or shivered as a dense evening fog crept into your bones, you know what weather can do to your defenses. It's un-pleasant, yes, but weather also makes for a useful tool in diagnosing illness.

At the time the *Nei Jing* was published in 200 BC, there were no EKG machines, no medical laboratories, no X-ray machines. The an-cient physicians had to rely on their observations of nature to make a diagnosis. And to a large extent, this is still true today.

If you experience dizziness during a heat wave, or chills and flu in the middle of a cold snap, it's easy to see that weather plays an inte-gral role in overall health. Even mild conditions—for example, a damp fog—can have consequences such as excess mucus and phlegm.

Once again, there are five culprits we can point to, five external climactic conditions—or *Devils*—that can attack our body-kingdom. These are **Heat, Cold, Dry, Damp,** and **Wind.** These devils can ap-pear on their own, or in combinations. Like strong emotions, any one of these can easily overpower our Wei Qi, and cause a storm within our body. To keep this from happening, we need to under-stand how each of these five devils affects our body-kingdom.

External Causes of Illness: The Heat Devil

Think about those hot sticky summer afternoons—when you just want to stop the world and float in a pool, sipping iced tea. This kind of weather isn't only uncomfortable, it can wreak havoc on your ner-vous system.

SIGNS OF HEAT

Red eyes	Delirium
Hot flashes	Disturbed sleep
Bright red complexion	Swollen glands
Excessive perspiration	Dark urine
Fever	Heat rash
Skin eruptions	Swollen joints
Fainting spells	Craving for cold, icy drinks

Even when it only lasts a few days, one-hundred-degree weather can be a formidable foe, causing high fevers, skin eruptions, headaches, and, most dangerously, a loss of body fluids. The Heart is the power center most sensitive to elevated temperatures, so if it becomes overheated, you may face troublesome behavioral symptoms, from fainting and palpitations to delirium and disturbed sleep.

STAY COOL WITH MUNG BEAN SOUP

YIELD: 4 TO 8 SERVINGS

INGREDIENTS:
1 POUND DRIED MUNG BEANS
8 CUPS WATER
SUGAR OR HONEY

Place the mung beans in a pot with the water and heat until boiling. Simmer for 2 hours, until the beans are softened. Add sugar or honey to taste. If suffering from skin problems, omit the sugar. Drink hot or cold during dry, hot weather
Mung beans are available at most Asian markets.

To avoid these symptoms, there are a number of things you can do during hot weather. Above all, avoid alcohol and spicy foods. They cause your core temperature to rise, an effect comparable to pouring gasoline on a fire.

It may seem self-evident, but try to stay in the shade and drink at least six glasses of water a day. Eat cooling foods, such as chilled, juicy vegetables and fruit (for example, cucumbers and tomatoes). These foods can act as an internal air conditioner, keeping your system cool and hydrated.

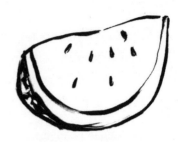

Watermelon: Cooling and Detoxifying

In China, watermelon has been used for centuries to cool the body and clean out toxins. When I was a child, summer didn't begin until the truck delivered a load of melons to our house. We looked forward to those first bites of the juicy red fruit. Little did I know that, years later, watermelon would actually save my life.

One day not long after graduation, I was interning at a Shanghai hospital when I nearly collapsed. I felt hot and achy, and I couldn't understand why. As it turned out, I had contracted a dangerous form of viral hepatitis, and soon found myself quarantined and confined to bed rest. I was given an IV and prescribed acupuncture and Chinese herbs. I was also put on a diet consisting of watermelons to reduce the fever and jaundice. The seeds help the Kidneys to function at their highest level and act as a diuretic, and the fruit and rind help to release Heat and toxins. After a month of who knows how many watermelons, the virus was beaten back, making this an excellent lesson in the healing power of a wonderful fruit.

External Causes of Illness: The Cold Devil

Say you've been working late. You pull into a supermarket on a cold winter evening to grab a quick salad. Since it's only a quick dash inside, you leave your coat in the backseat.

But as soon as your body contacts the icy air, the fluids inside begin to contract and stagnate, your muscles tighten to conserve energy, and in no time you begin to shiver. The Kidneys and the Bladder are the organs most vulnerable to a chill, so when the Cold Devil attacks, it seeps into your lower back, bladder, and genitals.

HEAT ME UP

Put 1/2 teaspoon of freshly ground pepper flakes on a plateful of hot noodles. It's a great way to head off a chill on a cool day.

The next morning you wake up and there it is, a head cold, a stiff back—possibly even a bladder infection. How did this happen so quickly? Think of it as a kind of perfect storm—the frigid air from the parking lot meeting the warmer temperature of your inner core, two weather fronts clashing inside your body. And if your defenses are already weak, the Cold Devil enters your kingdom even more swiftly, causing greater chaos.

SIGNS OF COLD

Pale, ashen complexion	Loss of endurance
Severe lower back pain	Craving for warm drinks
Impotence	Tendency to feel cold
Frigidity	Cold extremities: cold hands,
Loss of libido	cold feet
Prostate problems	Chronic cold weather illnesses
Fatigue	Brittle bones

How do you keep your Wei Qi strong and avoid the hazards of winter cold? Stay warm and dry, of course, but most of all, maintain a daily exercise regimen and a healthy diet that keeps your body physically and emotionally resilient. If you spend a lot of time in an air-conditioned environment, be on guard. Too much cold air while in a weakened state can penetrate your defenses and cause flu and colds.

There are other strategies you can use to stave off the cold weather. My flu-busting Chicken Soup, for instance (see page 98), or try an acupressure technique for sinusitis (see figure 3-11 on page 71), or some of the many common Chinese herbal cold remedies, such as Gan Mao Ling Tea. All can be used year-round to strengthen and clear your sinuses and protect your body.

External Causes of Illness: The Dry Devil

To understand the effects of dryness on the human body, imagine you are on a trip to the eastern corner of California. Picture yourself standing in a 140-mile-long former lakebed. The sandy earth is cracked and dry; the temperature is 130 degrees and rising. This barren landscape is called Death Valley.

While there, you might want to take a stroll. Yet after even a few swigs of water, the burning sun instantly makes you thirsty again. Your skin turns itchy and dry, your lips start to crack, and every breath sucks the moisture from your Lungs. This is an extreme version of what we call "dryness attacking your defensive shield." Almost instantaneously, your body loses vital fluids, creating a state of low energy and weakness.

SIGNS OF DRYNESS	
Dry, brittle hair and nails	Constipation
Dry mouth	Low urine
Dry nasal passages and sinuses	Lack of vaginal lubrication
Dry skin that wrinkles easily	Eczema
Dry irritated skin	Psoriasis
Dry cough	Dandruff
Tightness of chest	Dry, scaly pimples

This effect might come with the arid days of summer or from an autumn wind, but when dryness invades your kingdom, you usually feel the first symptoms through the skin. It can turn red and blister, or you might get a rash or patches of eczema. But if the dryness penetrates deeper and reaches the Lungs, the power center most sensitive to dryness, it can lead to a chronic cough, a possible precursor to asthma. If left unchecked, dryness can even reach the Lungs' partner organ, the Colon, resulting in cramps and constipation.

This condition is easily treated. If a patient is showing symptoms of chronic dryness, I will remoisturize with herbs and acupuncture. There are also several effective home remedies. Although it seems tempting, don't reach for that icy-cold soda; it's loaded with sugar and caffeine, and as you'll see in chapter 4, those ingredients are actually warming and drying, creating the opposite effect. Instead, try the Chinese way: drink a bowl of Mung Bean Soup (see page 34), or a glass of water with a tablespoon of honey and a teaspoon of lemon juice.

When the weather is hot and dry, it's also important to increase your protein intake. I recommend preparing a high protein meal such as my Easy Beef Stew (see page 278). Since your body is working harder to cool itself down, that extra protein will fortify your cells and Blood. Another healthy addition to your diet is raw vegetables and fruits, such as celery, cucumber, and apples, as well as the lubricating foods mentioned in chapter 4.

A humidifier or steam inhalation can also keep your respiratory passages moistened and lubricated. And, of course, the smartest way to stay healthy in an arid climate is to keep hydrated by drinking at least six to eight glasses of water each day.

External Causes of Illness: The Damp Devil

For many, living near a large body of water can be a lifelong dream. Lakes and oceans are beautiful, but those scenic vistas often come with a price—rain and moisture.

Consider a stubborn leak in the roof. The longer it rains, the wetter your carpet gets. Soon everything is a soggy mess, and nothing you do seems to stop the moisture from coming in.

Your body operates in the same way. When dampness attacks your kingdom and creeps into your castle window, it burrows deep into your power centers, making you feel heavy, swollen, and sluggish.

SIGNS OF DAMPNESS

Thick mucus in mouth, nose, and throat	Anorexia or bulimia
A tendency to bloat	Hemorrhoids
A tendency to gain weight and difficulty losing weight	Blood sugar disturbances
	Craving for sweets
Digestive issues: indigestion, abdominal pain, and excess stomach acid	Joint pain
	Fibroid tumors
	Varicose veins
Issues with obesity	Feelings of sluggishness and heaviness

Like an overflowing swamp, the body will produce a response to this dampness that the Chinese call *Tan*.

Tan is a hot and sticky phlegmlike substance that shows up in unpleasant ways: mucus in the throat and Lungs, loose and mushy stool, an oozing rash, lumps or cysts on the skin, perhaps even a tumor. Some people suffer water retention, bloating, chest congestion, nausea, and oily skin.

When I suspect a damp home environment, I ask my patient if there are any water or mold issues in the house. If so, it's a good idea to hire a specialist to inspect and remove the mold. By repairing stubborn leaks you are actively treating the causes of your Damp condition.

Acupuncture also helps, but first try limiting dairy products—these can lead to an accumulation of phlegm. And again, chapter 4 has some suggestions for easy, simple drying foods.

GOOD-BYE BLOATING WITH BARLEY AND RED BEAN SOUP

AN EXCELLENT FOOD TO SIP THROUGHOUT THE DAY.
YIELD: 8 TO 10 SERVINGS

INGREDIENTS:
8 OUNCES DRIED ADZUKI BEANS
8 OUNCES PEARL BARLEY
12 CUPS WATER
1/4 CUP SUGAR

Place the adzuki beans and barley in a pot and add water to cover. Soak overnight. In the morning, drain and place the adzuki beans and barley in a pot with the 12 cups of water. Bring to a boil. Lower the heat and simmer for 2 hours, then add the sugar. Pour into individual bowls and sip slowly, eating both the beans and liquid.

Barley and adzuki beans are an easy and natural way to eliminate unwanted fluids from the body. Adzuki beans are available at most Asian markets.

Sometimes, though, dampness can penetrate so deep that bones and joints are affected. Who hasn't heard elderly family members predicting the arrival of damp weather by the ache in their joints? If we leave these symptoms untreated, they can lead to a more chronic result of dampness, namely arthritis.

In China we call arthritis the *Bi syndrome*. Whenever I see achy joints, it tells me that your defensive energy (Wei Qi) has become weak. You have allowed atmospheric conditions to penetrate your body, obstructing the flow of energy and causing pain. If the arthritis is particularly sensitive to weather, it's likely you're suffering from Bi syndrome.

This condition has four varieties, each related to an extreme weather condition: *Hot Bi, Cold Bi, Damp Bi,* and *Windy Bi,* the Damp Bi condition being by far the most prevalent. Treatment for each involves relieving pain and boosting the Wei Qi.

External Causes of Illness: The Wind Devil

As each October rolls around the same thing happens. I'm suddenly flooded with calls from patients who aren't feeling well. My practice is located in an area where fall always brings powerful winds sweeping in from the desert, winds that can easily penetrate the body-kingdom and lead to fevers and skin problems. During this time I see a lot of boils, acne, and rashes—even nonspecific aches and pains that shift around the body.

And if patients have allowed the wind to penetrate deeper into their castle wall, it can affect their nervous system, causing trembling—even seizures.

SIGNS OF WIND	
Itching	Twitching
Dizziness	Numbness of limbs
Convulsions	Paralysis
Fever	Skin eruptions that move from
Muscle spasms	place to place
Stiffness of the head and neck	Aversion to wind
Vertigo	Sudden and rapid onset of
Tremors	symptoms

But hot winds are only part of the story. Icy winds, too, have their dangers, bringing on symptoms of cold and flu, as well as sore muscles and spasms.

Wind Qi does its damage by accessing your body at specific points on the shoulder and neck, as well as along the Gall Bladder meridian energy channel. Think of these points as entry ramps leading to destinations throughout your system. When Wind invades, it

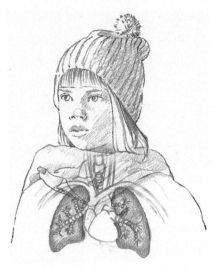

Protect the Lungs from the Cold Devil.

has a direct access to the muscles and tendons around your head and neck. This is why it's a good idea to always keep these areas covered and protected in a harsh wind.

If you suffer from a chronic stiff neck and muscular pain, rub some Red Flower Oil on the affected area. It's an effective treatment and is available in many health food stores.

The Five Devils illustrate exactly why we should be aware of weather and take care to protect ourselves. Although each Devil can pack quite a punch on its own, they often do their worst when they team up. And when combined with caustic emotions or internal weather, it's easy to see how disease can get a foothold.

The Internal Causes of Illness: The Five Emotions

Ancient Chinese physicians were keenly aware of the dangers our body faces—disease, infections, physical trauma—but they also suspected another cause of illness, one that lurked in the most unlikely of places: the boundless depths of human emotion.

Just as there are five major power centers, there are also five primary emotions that can lead to illness. They are *anger, sadness, joy, worry,* and *fear,* any of which can be enough to seriously disrupt your vital energy, or Qi, and weaken the immune system.

When Qi is flowing normally, it moves throughout the body by means of an intricate network of channels called *meridians* (see page 58). But physicians such as Dr. Sun Szu-miao (AD 590–682) and Dr.

Zhang Zi-he (1156–1228) discovered that when these emotions come on suddenly, or you simply hang on to them for too long, it upsets the energy flow through your meridians, making you sick.

The Emotional Roots of Illness

Picture yourself in line at the post office. It's ninety degrees and you've been waiting for a half hour. Suddenly, someone cuts into the line. When you try to protest, the person screams at you. You are now on the receiving end of an angry outburst. It's a fiery wave of emotional energy aimed directly at you, and it can continue to vibrate long after the incident has passed.

In a way, this wave is like a radio signal, and your body is acting like a giant receiver. When emotional outbursts are directed at you, the sound and emotional vibration are picked up and processed in the very heart of your power centers. Some people yell right back; others say nothing at all. One thing is for sure: Keeping these emotional "attacks" bottled up inside only adds to the collective heap of other negative experiences stored in your organs.

That's why unpleasant incidents like this are often followed by everything from a pounding heart to a whopping headache, even heart palpitations and panic attacks.

What happens if you lack the energy to withstand an assault like this? Your body gradually loses the ability to sort, separate, and release strong emotions. This can be disastrous, creating an angry volcano inside that leads to illness.

For me this was brought home in a very personal way.

An Overpowering Joy

Many years ago, China went through the Cultural Revolution, a difficult time for everyone. The rich were stripped of their homes and valuables, and many were forced into poverty and destitution. These were hard times, and hope was difficult to come by.

After many years, we Chinese were able to get back on our feet. But soon after, doctors began to notice something strange: an enormous rise in the rate of heart attacks.

It didn't make sense. Things were much better. Why were people getting sicker? The answer was right there in Chinese medicine.

Although conditions throughout China had greatly improved, malnutrition and stress had weakened many people's health. This became a big problem when the government returned their property and citizens were reunited with treasured possessions. The joy was so overwhelming that frail bodies had trouble processing these very strong emotions. In this state of heightened excitement, their rejuvenated Blood and increased Heat actually "exploded" blood vessels throughout the body, leading to a rash of heart attacks. This illustrates just how closely one's health is influenced by any emotion related to the Heart.

But this isn't the only organ affected by powerful events. As the *Nei Jing* teaches, each of the five power centers receives specific emotional frequencies and stores them in the body. Imagine then, the internal effect of an explosive verbal attack, especially when it is repeated over and over. No surprise that your defensive forces can gradually break down, losing the ability to keep illness at bay.

Your Emotional Weather

All of the five primary emotions have the ability to attack your power centers from within. They also create their own atmospheric conditions *inside* the body. The best way to understand this is to picture a host of powerful weather systems moving through your energy channels. If these emotional systems become strong or frequent enough, they create storms that can ravage your body in a number of ways.

EMOTION	INTERNAL CLIMATE
Joy	Heat
Anger	Wind, Fire, Heat
Fear	Cold
Worry	Dampness
Sadness	Dryness

My job is to predict and analyze these weather patterns and provide a treatment that will prevent them from returning. To do this I need to target the emotions for these disturbances.

- Extremes of **joy, excitement,** and **agitation** create an explosive, internal **Heat wave.**
- Chronic **anger** and **frustration** produce a turbulent **Wind,** as well as volcanic **Fire** and **Heat.**
- Excessive **fear** slows and constricts bodily functions, creating a **Cold front.**
- Daily **worry and anxiety** causes your digestive organs to become sluggish and **Damp.**
- Continual **sadness** and **grief** leads to dehydration and **Dry spells.**

Let's look at each of the five primary emotions and the internal weather they create.

Joy: Internal Heat

Seeing what the Heart can do makes it easier to understand why it is the organ most attuned to the frequencies of **joy** and **passion**. When balanced, joy is a positive emotion that keeps your kingdom happy and at peace. But joy and excitement can also spin out of control, leading to overstimulation of the Heart energy network. Under these

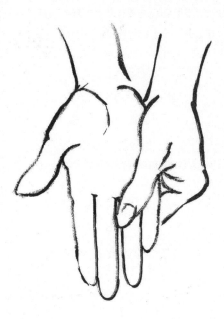

Figure 2-2. Massage your hands between fourth and fifth fingers to alleviate stress.

conditions, good feelings actually become the enemy, turning this organ into a raging furnace and creating an explosive inner Heat. In this state, it's easy to suffer disturbed sleep and confused thought patterns. Worse symptoms such as skin eruptions, uneven blood pressure, and even heart attacks can follow.

A good way to ease these symptoms is with my Heart Massage (see figure 3-3 on page 64). As soon as you start feeling agitated, try massaging your hands, especially the fourth and fifth fingers (see figure 2-2). Also, try the Heart Lock-In technique (page 301), and take a look at some of the seasonal foods for the Heart (page 214).

Sadness: Internal Dryness

When you receive vibrations of grief and sadness, the organ most affected is your mighty queen, the Lungs. Too many people harbor feelings of sadness, burying them for long periods of time. Gradually, repressing these feelings will slow your queen's function, leading to symptoms from internal dryness to the pores in your skin closing up. Since the nose is the gateway to the Lungs, you might also experience chronic bronchitis, sinusitis, dry skin, and dehydration.

As I've mentioned in earlier chapters, if I suspect my patients are bottling up their grief and sadness, I usually add some simple advice to the prescription: rent a sad movie and let the tears flow! There's nothing like a good cry to release those toxic pent-up feelings. I also recommend appropriate foods such as Soothing Pear Skin Tea for the Lungs (see page 219), or ask them to try my daily organ exercises; in particular, massaging the web joint between thumb and index finger (see figure 3-5 on page 65). Another good remedy is a breathing meditation for the Lungs (see page 79).

By cracking the top off those bottled emotions, you drain away the effects from whatever event caused them, interrupting the dangerous influence on the Heart and other organs.

Anger: Internal Fire, Wind, Heat

One of the strongest of all emotions, anger is picked up most easily by the commander of your Blood, the Liver.

Think of what it's like to be young. Emotions are raw and anger and frustration are easily expressed. Sit beside a baby on an airplane and you'll know when the cabin pressure is driving it crazy. By releasing its stress, the baby is letting you know exactly how it feels. And when its discomfort is gone, there's that smile again. The fact that kids can bounce back so quickly means that their Qi is flowing, and they are flexible and resilient.

With age, people tend to lose this flexibility.

It's been a long day, and as you leave the office, the boss yells at you for losing an e-mail. On the way home, the creeping traffic comes to a stop. Inside your body-kingdom, the dragon of stress begins to stir. You beat the steering wheel and scream at the car next to you, while inside your body excessive Heat rushes to your head, causing vessels to constrict. Suddenly a city bus cuts you off and all at once the vital flow of Blood is strangled, disrupting the even tempo your system needs to function smoothly. In no time you're suffering a thundering headache—and for an unlucky few, possibly something worse.

Repeating this cycle over and over, day after day, for years on end, can send your Liver into a complete burnout mode. With enough time, these spikes of negative emotion will fry your internal electrical system, leaving the Liver overtaxed and prone to disease. This is precisely when your body begins to experience serious conditions such as chronic fatigue, heart attacks, substance abuse, and even cancer.

It's a good illustration of why we need to create appropriate ways of expressing our frustration and stress, and keep the Liver working together in a harmonious relationship.

Worry: Internal Dampness

Unless you live in a cabin deep in the forest, the challenges of modern life are never far away. It's not hard to find yourself anxious and worried, and when that happens it's the Stomach and Spleen that are affected. As the primary organs in charge of metabolism and digestion, they are far more susceptible to emotions of anxiety and worry.

When your power centers are balanced, you are able to express worries to others in a clear and reasonable way. A constant state of anxiety, however, causes your Stomach and Spleen to break down. They lose the ability to properly receive nutrients and create enough Blood and Qi. Eventually, these anxious feelings become "stuck" to those organs, leading to a host of troublesome symptoms: fatigue, dull headaches, water retention, chronic stomachaches, weight gain, as well as fluctuations in blood sugar.

Along with herbs and acupuncture, you can treat a weak Spleen by massaging your digestive organs before you eat (see figure 2-4). By massaging your digestive organs and their corresponding energy channels, you activate Blood and Qi and stimulate the digestive process. Another effective therapy is a daily meditation for the digestive organs (see page 137). This condition always improves with the right food in moderation. Don't skip meals; and do stick to high-energy foods, such as protein soups and stews, and root vegetables, such as squash and sweet potatoes.

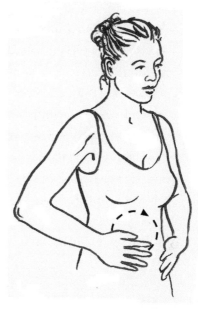

Figure 2-4. Massage your digestive organs in a clockwise motion before you eat.

Fear: Internal Cold

Fear is probably more damaging to the body than any of the other five emotions. Unfortunately, it's also part of daily life. It can hit anywhere. When that wayward pedestrian pops out in front of your moving car, your heart pounds, you gasp for breath, your body freezes up. Even though you stop the car in time, you may start to shiver with fright. This is a perfect example of fear attacking your kingdom.

I recently observed this myself when my granddaughter suddenly fell off her bike. Luckily she wasn't hurt. But despite the hot summer weather, she began shivering uncontrollably. The emotion of fear and Cold had attacked her kingdom, and did not let go until we

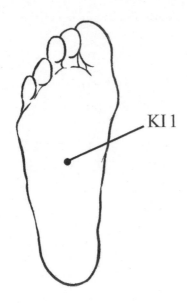

KI 1

Figure 2-5. Press acupoint *Kidney 1* to strengthen the Kidneys and recharge your batteries.

wrapped her in warm blankets and took her home to rest.

Whenever you experience these feelings of terror, they are picked up and stored in your kingdom's ministry of power, the Kidneys. It doesn't matter where the fear comes from— a dangerous episode, personal abuse; if the event is sudden and explosive, it constricts and shuts off the energy flow to and from this organ. When your Kidneys are strong and healthy, you can process these jolts. You can also better sustain periods of prolonged fear.

But if, like my granddaughter, you are unable to process your fears, or you don't know how, it can leave your Kidneys open to attack. When I see physical symptoms related to the Kidneys, such as seizures, stiff joints, bladder issues, and infertility, they are usually signs of hidden and unprocessed fear. I treat these symptoms accordingly, but I also recommend having a close group of family and friends for support. People who can help you through a fearful period can often make an enormous difference in how your body processes this strong emotion.

Finally, doing some daily internal organ exercises along the meridians helps to strengthen the Kidneys, especially at the small of the back and the bottom of your feet (see figure 2-5). This works because these points are directly connected to the Kidneys and their energy channels (see figure 3-17 on page 77). Foods such as miso soup, walnuts, black beans, figs, and dates are also highly beneficial for your ministry of power.

To prevent these emotional weather fronts from affecting your kingdom, tune in and listen to your body. Stay vigilant, and try not to let situations and events determine the emotional load your body takes on.

By allowing these attackers to find a way past your defensive forces, you are leaving your leadership open to the storms of disease and illness. As we'll see in the next section, these emotional influences on the *inside*, combined with temperature changes sent from the *outside*, often lead to the biggest health challenges of all.

A Clash of Outer Climate, Inner Climate: Tracy

Last winter, Tracy came into my office complaining of severe tinnitus (ringing) in both ears. She had already seen a number of doctors, who had given her medication for her symptoms. But recently the ringing had returned full force. After examining her, I suspected that two different weather systems were behind this. Through a pulse diagnosis (see pages 248–253), I detected a blockage, an internal Wind caused by emotion that was leading to Heat and stress. As it happens, there had also been a cool October breeze blowing all week.

I knew that some sort of emotional Heat was clashing with the Cold wind, creating an energy blockage in her ear. This is possible because the Liver and Gall Bladder are connected by energy channels located on the inside of the ear canal (see figure 3-12 on page 72).

Sure enough, Tracy confided that her tinnitus had returned at the same time that her best friend had become gravely ill. She had also recently exchanged angry phone calls with her son.

I began by treating the points along her Gall Bladder, Liver, and Kidney channels. By using acupuncture, herbs, and relaxation techniques, we were able to free the blockage and cure the ringing. She recently told me that since the treatment, she has become more open and understanding of past events. She has resolved the issues with her family, and is enjoying a newfound peace.

When storms like these attack from both within and without, it's necessary to take action and treat the causes, before a simple symptom becomes a health crisis of much larger proportions.

Viruses and Pathogens

There is another cause of disease, one that is beyond anyone's control: the invisible microbes that make up viruses, pathogens, and bacteria. Western medicine meets these organisms with flu shots or man-made antibiotics, but through the centuries the Chinese have developed a specialized arsenal of natural antiviral and antibacterial herbs to treat these conditions (see page 233). These herbs not only target and eliminate the pathogen; they strengthen and nourish the immune system to withstand future bacterial and viral attacks.

Although you can't always avoid viruses, here are precautions you can take: Stay warm in the winter months, avoid stressful emotions, and keep your environment as germ free as possible.

FIRST VACCINE

The Chinese discovered an herbal formula for smallpox in 1713, predating Western medicine by more than fifty years.

The Miscellaneous Causes of Illness: Unforeseen Events

When people think of disease, they usually don't take into account one of the most obvious causes: injury. It can happen so quickly: a ladder collapses underneath you, or your son's bike sends you sprawling. Accidents happen, and when they result in an unexpected physical injury, the effect on your health can be profound.

Let's say you reach into the oven and badly burn your arm. The event itself is startling, and painful, so much so that a jolt is sent through your energy system. Inside your channels an instant blockage is created, or what we call a "congestion of Qi."

This blockage can attack the body just like any virus, or icy wind. And the condition only becomes more acute when you react to the accident with fear, anger, or worry. These intense emotional vibrations congest the Qi further, weakening your power centers and opening up your body to disease and illness. Unfortunately, I have seen this malicious cause and effect many times in my practice.

Accidents to Insights: Brian

The day Brian hobbled into my office last year, he was in great pain and deeply depressed. When I asked him why, the story he told me was nothing short of astonishing.

Four months earlier, Brian had been rushing to catch the bus for his morning commute. He had just put his foot on the step to climb aboard when the bus driver, who wasn't paying attention, closed the door, trapping his foot inside. As horrified onlookers watched, the bus drove off, dragging Brian down the street. For sixty sickening seconds he scraped along the pavement, just inches from one of the bus's wheels. Finally, the driver braked for traffic and Brian struggled free. The bus driver, however, was unaware that Brian was lying underneath the bus, and sped on. Despite severe trauma to his head, neck, and pelvis, Brian rolled away from the rear wheels, a split second before the bus would have crushed him.

Brian was alive but his injuries were critical. Doctors diagnosed him with a severe concussion. Every vertebra in his body was out of alignment, and his lumbar disk had completely disintegrated.

For months, the hospital treated his shock and trauma with drugs and physical therapy, but his pain remained excruciating. Desperate for something that could help, he called my office and made an appointment.

A few months of treatment followed, and Brian began to see results almost immediately. "I felt better so quickly," he recounted. "Not only was I healing, but I was concentrating better than I ever had. My thoughts were coming into focus and I was sleeping well again. Strange as it seems, I also experienced a number of positive side effects from my treatment. My energy has actually increased. I've lost weight, and I'm growing hair on my head in places that have been bald for years. Best of all, my lifelong battle with depression is gone. Acupuncture has truly given me a new life."

What happened to Brian? Because of his accident, he experienced a violent "congestion of Qi." This resulted in extensive blockages along his Kidneys, Liver, Bladder, and Gall Bladder channels. In addition to the injuries sustained during his accident, these blockages were perpetuating his pain.

The only way Brian was going to get better was to clear this energy gridlock. Acupuncture needles work a lot like a tow truck, unblocking your energy traffic jams. By precisely targeting and removing blockages of Qi, acupuncture frees the energy, moves the Blood, and best of all, releases pain.

With a few gentle needles, I was not only able to unblock the fear and pain in Brian's Kidney and Bladder channels, but also managed to remove years of preexisting stagnation and depression in his Liver channels.

Tuning in and Taking Charge

Now that you have begun to learn how Chinese medicine understands the major causes of illness, it's time to start connecting the dots.

As you can see, for the Chinese practitioner, the causes of illness come in many guises: a hot wind, an angry family member, or an icy office cubicle. All are powerful enemies that, when combined, make up a dangerous army attacking our body-kingdom's defenses.

Rather than looking at aches, pains, flu, and other illness as random events, the next time you get sick, ask yourself these questions: Was there an emotional trigger to your illness? Did you get caught outside in extreme weather? If you suffered an injury, are you relying solely on medication, or are you helping your immune system to heal in other ways? Understanding how you became ill is the biggest step to discovering the cure.

Ahead, we'll look at the fourth common cause of illness: lifestyle factors. We'll investigate positive diet, exercise, and lifestyle habits, all behaviors that are pivotal in preventing physical and emotional trauma. Only by learning how to create a balanced lifestyle can you build a strong immune system—a vital Wei Qi that will always be there to guard your kingdom.

DR. TING'S TOTAL HEALTH ESSENTIALS

YIN AND YANG

Both must coexist peacefully to maintain good health.

- **Yin** is a colder, passive, static energy.
- **Yang** is an active, fiery energy.

4 Basic Forms of Qi

- Original Qi, or Jing Qi
- Gu Qi
- Da Qi
- Shen Qi

The 4 Causes of Disease

- **Internal:** emotions, psychological trauma
- **External:** viruses, pathogens
- **Miscellaneous:** injuries, accidents, natural disasters
- **Lifestyle:** overwork, poor diet, social habits, inappropriate or lack of exercise (these will be discussed in later chapters)

External Causes of Illness: The 5 Weather Devils

- Heat Devil
- Cold Devil
- Dry Devil
- Damp Devil
- Wind Devil

Internal Causes of Illness: The 5 Major Emotions

Each of your five power centers receives specific emotional frequencies and stores them in your body.

- Joy
- Anger
- Fear
- Worry
- Sadness

3

Move and Breathe
Building Your Internal Qi

When I was a young child in China, I was thin, sickly, and very shy. Gym class was not exactly one of my strengths, so it was a surprise when I came to class one day to find that my schoolmates had elected me president of the elementary student council. At the time, this job had one main function: to lead the entire school in a daily series of mandatory exercises called Guang Bo. My classmates thought it was hysterical to put me in charge of these exercises, especially after I had fainted in the middle of my school's eight-hundred-meter dash!

But each morning I was given the bullhorn, and we all marched out to the school square. For twenty minutes I led hundreds of students with my tiny, shrill voice, all the while bending, stretching, and lunging. My classmates teased me mercilessly, but I kept at it. It was my job and I was not going to give up, even if I did sound like a mouse.

Little did I know that the exercises we did in that small school square would be the first step in creating a constant flow of Qi within our young bodies. Since then I've come to appreciate the importance of building and cultivating the flow of Qi on a daily basis.

Often my patients will come into my office and tell me they come home after work feeling sluggish and depressed. My answer is always the same. It's because they've been sitting all day and concentrating. Their energy is used up and their Qi reserves are down. Naturally, they feel wiped out.

When Qi is stagnant or moving slowly, not only does it leave the door open for physical health to deteriorate, but your emotions and mental health also take a dive. Parking your body behind a desk or steering wheel only cuts you off from natural energy flow. Qi needs to move to ward off illness and help you feel your best.

The Meridians: Your Highways of Qi

Thousands of years ago, Chinese physicians discovered that Qi runs along fourteen channels, or *meridians*, throughout the body. Think of them as superhighways of energy: seven energy channels running along the front of your body, and seven along the back.

Like an interstate highway that stretches from city to city, each meridian is coupled or connected to one of your five major power centers. For example, one meridian connects to the king, your Heart. Other highways lead from the Liver, the Gall Bladder, and so on. Where do all these highways end up? After passing through your internal organs, they surface on the outside of your body, where they are accessible as acupuncture and acupressure points.

A lot of people think pain and illness are mysterious events that lodge in their body, but the cause is nothing more than a traffic jam along one of these energy highways.

Just like that interstate, each meridian has its own set of on and off ramps. A total of 365 points along these energy channels access your individual meridians and power centers.

To keep your body healthy and strong, the Qi must move uninterruptedly throughout these meridians. The quality of the food you eat, the stability of your emotional health, and the cleanliness of the air you breathe are all vital to keeping these channels open and free.

Even under the best conditions, however, illness can still strike. Qi can be choked off due to physical or emotional distress, causing a debilitating blockage. I call it "Qi gridlock." This "traffic" congestion shows up in the form of sinus pain, or maybe achy joints or a headache. As a Chinese physician, I sometimes think of myself as a highway patrol officer clearing that accident and getting the highway moving again. To treat these internal blockages, I access the meridian highways using a variety of treatments, such as a gentle needling technique called acupuncture, or with a personalized formula of herbs.

When the meridians are flowing as they should, your muscles and organs stay strong, allowing you to radiate a healthy energy vibration. Keeping your emotions even and under control leads to better decisions and makes it easier to react more calmly to life's ups and downs.

Naturally, body movement and exercise are key ingredients to your health and your life. The movement that you create on the outside is essential to keeping your Qi network moving freely and easily on the inside.

Professional athletes are a great example. They tend to be extraordinarily measured and calm, even if they are thrown unexpected obstacles. Take Lance Armstrong, for instance. During one of the most grueling events, the ninth stage of the 2003 Tour de France, Armstrong swerved to avoid a downed rider, Joseba Beloki, who had locked

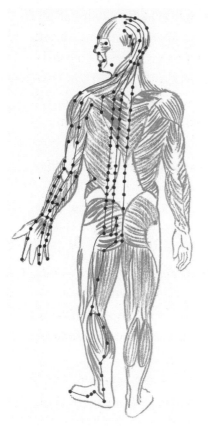

Figure 3-1. Acupuncture Points on the Body

up his wheel on a melted road surface. Many athletes would have fallen, but Armstrong managed to veer off into a nearby field. Miraculously, he pedaled through the dirt, hopped the embankment, and caught up with the pack at the bottom of the hill, going on to win the stage. Yes, his physical condition played a big role, but his miraculous save would not have been possible unless his Qi network was operating at the highest level. This is the surest way to stay alert, focused, and able to overcome any obstacle.

Building Qi from the Inside Out

When I was young we had little time for team sports or extracurricular programs. After school, there was always lots chores to do, and without electrical appliances, my brothers and sisters and I were required to boil our water for cooking and washing. Because I grew up during World War II and the Cultural Revolution, there were times when we weren't getting the right foods, or enough of them to compensate for all the energy we were using. Consequently my immune system was greatly weakened, opening up my body to serious physical illnesses and emotional trauma.

It's not surprising that many years later, when I came to live in the United States, I was still very weak. I had already survived cancer, diphtheria, and tuberculosis. But now I found myself in a completely foreign country with few friends or family.

I had come to the United States to start my own practice and bring Chinese medicine to as many people as I could, and that meant having stamina. I first needed to work for my sponsor family, take English lessons, and prepare for my U.S. acupuncture certification exams. To accomplish all of these things, I had to get stronger. Because I understood Chinese medicine, I knew it was time to cultivate my inner energy network to create a larger reserve to draw from. I had to start from the inside and work out.

Thinking back on those childhood exercises I did in the school square, I decided the best way to build up this inner energy network was to start a simple daily routine. The first step was to get the Qi flowing consistently, at an even pace, so my immune system could rebuild itself.

I spent the next ten years designing and perfecting my own personal organ and meridian exercise routine. These exercises are based on Chinese medical theory, as well as a series of movements found in selected Chinese martial arts traditions.

I've been using them daily for the last twenty years, and I can honestly say that I'm healthier and stronger now than I have ever been. These exercises are especially designed to stimulate a consistent flow of energy through the meridians and power centers, and are probably the most important form of preventative medicine you can possibly do.

Esther Ting's Internal Organ and Meridian Exercises

Your head, hands, arms, ears, legs, and feet all have pressure points that are nestled along your energy highways and lead directly to your five power centers. Think of them as the gateways to your cardiac, respiratory, and digestive organs.

By touching individual points along the *outside* of your meridians, you are helping to remove blockages occurring on the *inside* of your body. This has the effect of strengthening your immune system, increasing concentration, and even soothing depression. Best of all, this twenty-minute exercise routine is suitable for all ages, anytime, anywhere. You can even try them on your pets!

My internal organ exercise is divided into three parts, each of which has three steps, making for nine distinct phases of the exercise. Don't worry—each takes only about two minutes.

Incorporating the meridian massage into your daily routine means you are practicing the best form of preventative medicine there is. No expensive doctor's visits or medication! The vitality you create goes beyond muscle strength, giving you an inner strength that lasts.

How They Work

The first group of exercises (parts 1–3) uses a gentle finger and foot massage that directly stimulates your kingdom's five Zhang power centers. By targeting specific points on your hands and feet, you are sending healing energy to your Liver, Heart, Kidneys, Lungs, and Spleen, as well their accompanying Fu organs (see chapter 1).

In the second group (parts 4–5), you add slightly more force, with a gentle patting motion along the entire length of your body. The aim is to increase the circulation along the entire meridian system, and really get it flowing.

In the last group (part 6), you'll end with some soothing breathing exercises. This not only helps to physically move the Qi but also enhances Blood supply and circulation.

With each exercise you will cycle through your meridians and organs two to three times, giving your Qi a full workout. If at any point during your day you are feeling tense, nervous, or anxious, these exercises are a wonderful way to calm and balance your system.

In my experience, performing these exercises in the morning works best, but you can try them at other times of the day as well. Best of all, you don't have to visit a gym. They can be done on the floor, while sitting at the office, or between household chores. Every time you stimulate and massage your meridians and their points, you are activating your organs to work more efficiently for you.

Part One
The Power Centers in Your Hands: Easy Relief for Tension, Insomnia, and Pain

Remember kindergarten? You probably spent hours playing with a ball of clay or some Silly Putty. Think about massaging your pressure points in exactly the same way. Gently knead and press the following points until the Qi flows.

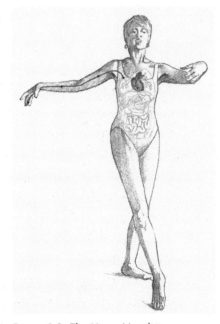

Hand and Finger Massage

Step One: Start by rubbing your hands together briskly. Now hold your left palm up (see figure 3-3), and put your right thumb on top and your right index finger on the bottom of your palm. Use that

Figure 3-2. The Heart Meridian

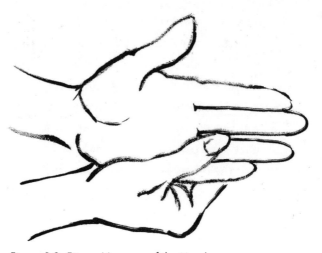

Figure 3-3. Finger Massage of the Hands

thumb to gently knead your way up to the tip of your little finger. Do the same for each finger this way until you have massaged your whole hand.

What exactly does all this pulling and stretching do? By kneading your *pinkie, ring finger,* and *middle fingers,* you are massaging the arteries and organs along the various energy channels that protect the Heart (see figure 3-2). If you're feeling nervous before asking for a raise, or singing a church solo, massage your wrist crease at acupoints *Heart 7, Pericardium 6,* and *Pericardium 8* to calm you down. These are also good points for nausea and insomnia (see figure 3-4).

Thumbs can be pressed and kneaded in the same way, directly benefiting the Lungs. The same is true for the index finger, which soothes and benefits the Colon. If you're constipated, try rubbing thumb and index finger a few times a day to relieve the condition.

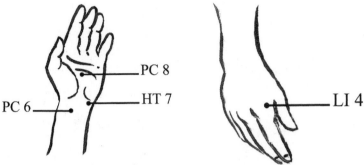

Figure 3-4. Acupressure Points for
Tension and Stress   Figure 3-5. Acupoints for Pain and Stress

Massaging the web between the thumb and index finger is often
used for general pain relief (*Large Intestine 4*) (see figure 3-5).

Step Two: Now, flip your hand use your thumb and index finger
to repeat the entire process on the back of the hand. When you're
done, repeat the entire massage (steps one and two) on your right
palm, using your left thumb in exactly the same way.

Step Three: When all the pressure points have been massaged,
take a moment to rub and soothe the back of your hands. Then let
both wrists relax.

Shake them out ten times to open up the meridians in the wrists
and let the energy flow.

Part Two
The Power Centers in Your Feet: Maximize Your
Energy, and Massage Away Stress and Indigestion

Let's face it; most of us take our feet for granted. We stuff them into
shoes that are too small, or stand on them for hours at a time. But
did you know that your feet are the gateway to six major meridian

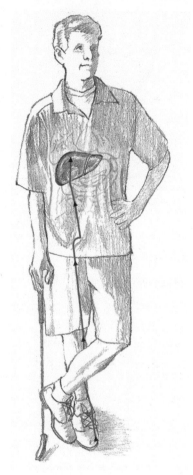

Figure 3-6. The Liver Meridian

channels—the Stomach, Spleen, Liver, Gall Bladder, Kidneys, and Bladder?

Think about it. Six superhighways leading from your feet to a different destination. You'll find that the big toe is a direct road to the Liver meridian (see figure 3-6). As you now know, the Liver commands many of your emotions, including stress and anger. It is also in charge of your strategy and focus. By massaging your big toes, you will not only help balance your emotions, but you will find it easier to remain calm and centered.

And that's just your big toes. Other meridians run along the left and right side of your toes and ankles. If you are suffering from corns, bunions, and/or painful feet, it could be due to pinched meridians.

That's why I always advise my patients to start with the foot massage.

Foot Massage

Step One: Sitting comfortably, cross your right foot over your left thigh, and let it rest there (see figure 3-7). Now rub the bottom of your foot vigorously until it warms up. This simple motion sends energy to your Spleen and Stomach, as well as your Kidneys.

If you are suffering from indigestion, take the opportunity to massage the Achilles tendon, under the heel, as well as the outside edge of the big toe. This area connects directly to the Spleen, and helps to strengthen your digestion.

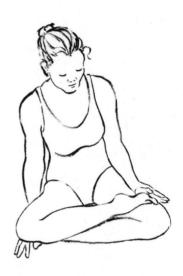

If you're experiencing fatigue or loss of energy, gently massage the balls of your feet. This directly accesses the Kidney meridian, which leads to your ministry of power. The channel starts under the small toe and extends across the ball of the foot, up the inside of your leg to your collarbone.

Now, placing your thumb on the bottom of your foot, and your index finger on the top, massage from the heel to the tip of your big toe, using the same

Figure 3-7. Foot Massage

pressure you used on your hand. Continue this exercise until each of your toes is fully massaged. Then turn the foot over and massage the top of the foot from the ankle to the tip of each toe, starting with your big toe and finishing with your pinkie.

Step Two: Next, turn your foot over and find a spot on the top of your foot. We'll call this **point one** (*Liver 2*). Rub this area well. Then, using your thumbs, press the joint directly an inch *below* your big toe and second toe. We'll call it **point two** (*Liver 3*) (see figure 3-8). Yes, this joint can be sensitive, but don't be afraid to push hard. These two points are connected to your Liver; massaging here can alleviate a lot of stress and anxiety. Press again, then interchange between each of these points ten times apiece.

Now for **point three** (*Stomach 44*). It's located on the joint between the second and third toe. This point sends energy to the Stomach and Spleen. It eases digestion and is another good way to reduce anxiety and worry. **Point four** (*Gall Bladder 43*) is located

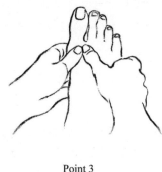

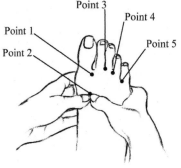

Figure 3-8. Foot Points

underneath the fourth toe, and by massaging here, you are helping your Gall Bladder stay healthy and fit. **Point five** (*Bladder 67*) is the joint directly underneath the pinkie, and targets the Bladder.

Start at point one and press each of these five points in quick succession. As you work toward the little toe, your thumb should press on top, while the index finger naturally presses from below.

Step Three: Repeat the entire sequence on the opposite foot.

Now that the Qi is surging to the Kidneys, Lungs, Liver, Heart, and Stomach, you should feel more refreshed, and ready to move on to the final stage.

Part Three
The Power Centers in Your Head: Soothe Headaches, Increase Vision, and Relieve Sinus Congestion

Your Face

In Chinese medicine, the face is a very powerful place in the body. Not only does it reveal a great deal about a person's inner health, but it is also the beginning and end of numerous energy highways.

Massaging your face *above* the eyes directly targets a number of major power centers and their related organs, including the Large Intestine and the Bladder.

Facial Massage

Step One: Start by placing the knuckles of your index finger on the inner eyebrow (see figure 3-9). Smooth and stretch the brow outward *above* your eye until you reach your temples. Now move your knuckles *below* the eyes to the bridge of the nose and smooth outward underneath the eye until you again reach your temples.

Massaging the area around your eyes is not only good for your vision, but it clears your head and relieves headaches. Since the Liver rules the eyes and also manages emotions of anger and frustration, a quick massage after an argument can literally smooth away that anger.

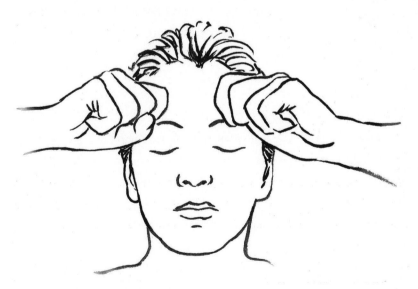

Figure 3-9. Inner Eyebrow Massage

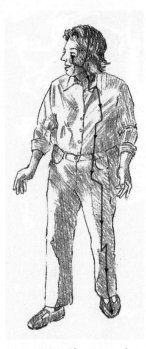

Figure 3-10. The Stomach
Meridian is one of the few
meridians that end in the
face.

Step Two: The area *below* your eyes targets your Stomach meridians (see figure 3-10), as well as your Lungs and Colon. Massaging under the eyes is good for sinus infections as well as indigestion.

To access it, place your flattened palms on the sides of your temples, stretching the skin tight. Remember, this entire movement counts as one movement. Massage these three areas—eyebrow, under eye, temples—in quick succession.

Do this gentle knuckle massage six times.

Step Three: Finish your facial massage by sweeping the contours of your face with your palms, from your temples to your chin. Pressing the cheeks gives energy to the Heart. Pressure to the forehead strengthens the Kidneys and Bladder.

This movement is also repeated six times.

Your Nose

The next few exercises are especially helpful for relieving sinus congestion during allergy season, as well as to help ward off colds and flu. The series consists of pressing four points.

Nose and Sinus Massage

Step One: First, begin by using your index or middle fingers to press the **first point** (*Large Intestine 20*) along the base of your nose (see

figure 3-11). Since nostrils are the
entry point for the air you breathe,
this directly affects the Lungs,
Colon, and, of course, the nose
and sinus cavities.

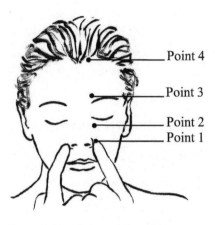

Step Two: The **second point**
(Stomach 1) is located beside the
bridge of the nose. Pressing here
increases energy flow to the Stomach and Spleen.

Step Three: The **third point**
(Gall Bladder 14) is on the inner
eyebrow.

Figure 3-11. Nose and Sinus Massage

Step Four: Rubbing the temples vigorously increases blood flow
to your scalp and brain.

Touch each of these three points in a simple progression for
about a second apiece.

Once again, perform a set of six.

Your Scalp

Let's say it's a long Friday and you're facing an hour of heavy com-
muting before you get home. You're tired and you don't know how
you'll make it. Here is a quick massage that will help clear that sluggish energy and keep you mentally sharp. Some of my patients will
even do this before a speaking engagement or presentation.

Scalp Massage

Step One: First, using the tips of your fingers, massage your scalp
from front to back, ten times. This movement helps to energize the

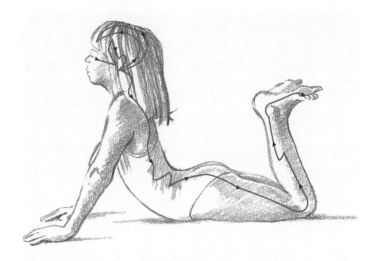

Figure 3-12. The Gall Bladder Meridian

scalp and enriches the Blood flowing to the brain. Then, using your full palm, press those knobby bumps at the base of your skull, ten times. This gentle motion stimulates the Gall Bladder channel (see figure 3-12), a meridian that happens to be one of the longest in the entire body. It starts in the foot and travels all the way up to the scalp, crisscrossing it several times. If you feel a headache coming on, massage this area vigorously. It is also a helpful area to stimulate hair growth.

Step Two: Now let's move to your ears. Since your ears are connected to every meridian in the body, rubbing them gives your entire body a gentle massage. It's simple: Just rub ten times from top to bottom.

Step Three: Ever wonder why stress makes you get a stiff neck? It's because the Gall Bladder highway travels right through this area.

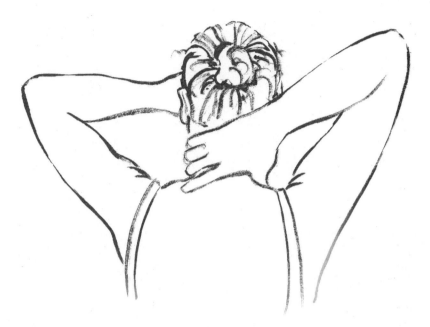

Figure 3-13. Neck Massage

To massage it properly, it's best to stabilize everything by holding your forehead. This relaxes the spinal column and central nervous system. Support the front of your forehead with your left hand, while squeezing the back of your neck with your right hand (see figure 3-13). Do this ten times. Now reverse your hands and repeat the process ten times.

You have now finished the first section of my exercises. By massaging your hands, feet, head, ears, and face, you have directly strengthened each of your five power centers. You should feel more refreshed and energized. Now it's time to get your meridian highways moving and flowing.

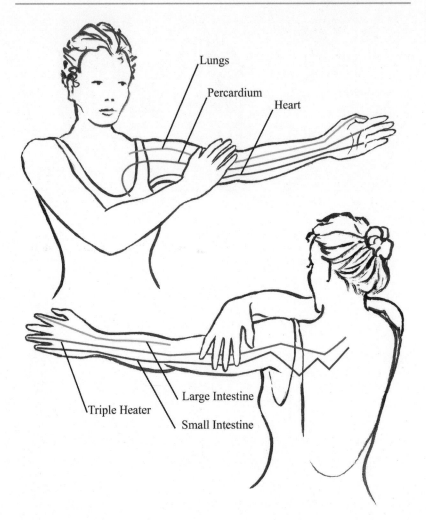

Figure 3-14. Meridians in the Arms

Part Four
Strengthening the Meridians in Your Upper Body

As you know, your meridian channels run throughout your body. They break down like this: There are six major highways in your upper body: three along the outside of your arms and three on the inner side (see figure 3-14). This time, instead of pressing specific points, you are going to sweep along this entire meridian system and give it a significant boost.

Upper Body Patting Exercise

Step One: Begin by standing with your feet shoulder-width apart. Extend your left arm straight out, in front of you, and use the palm of your right hand to gently pat inside and outside your extended hand and arm. Now extend your right arm and repeat, using your left hand to do the patting (see figure 3-14).

When done, relax by swinging your arms loosely for a count of seven.

Step Two: Next, make a fist with both hands and reach around your sides to your back. Pat upward from the buttocks to the shoulder blades, along both sides of the spine. The particular meridian you're targeting

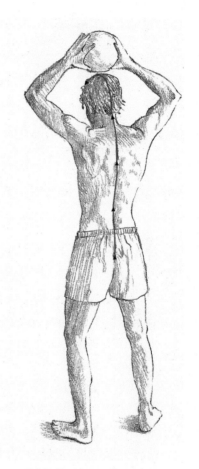

Figure 3-15. Du Mai or Governing Vessel

is one of two superhighways called the *Du Mai*, or Governing Vessel meridians. It is the main traffic artery, or energy circuit, along your back and spine. It also intersects with the Bladder meridian, giving a major boost to your ministry of power (see figures 3-15 and 3-18). Several minor highways also merge on and off the Governing Vessel. This makes it one of the most powerful points in your entire body, so make sure to do this exercise series seven times.

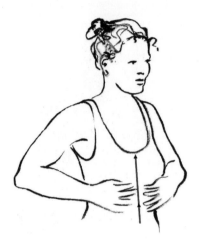

Figure 3-16. Massaging the Conception Vessel

Now you'll stimulate the highways along the front of your body.

Step Three: Start by moving your right hand across your body to the upper left side and patting all the way down your left side, from shoulder to groin. This exercise stimulates the flow of energy throughout the Stomach and Spleen meridians, helping to strengthen your metabolism and digestion. Do this motion seven times, then change hands and repeat seven times on the right side of your body. Please note that men should pat the entire length of the chest, whereas women should skip the area over the breast.

Step Four: Finally, with both hands, pat down the center of your chest in a straight line from your breastbone to your abdomen (see figure 3-16). This helps boost your Heart and your thymus gland, enhancing both circulation and energy. It also strengthens the *Ren Mai*, or Conception Vessel Meridian (figure 3-17), that major energy highway along the front of the body.

Again, do these chest pats for a count of seven.

If you are gassy, bloated, or constipated, try this bonus exercise: Place your hands on your abdomen and pat it like a drum.

Part Five
Strengthening the Meridians in Your Lower Body

Your legs support your weight and motivate you around the world. They also contain the four major meridians that run from the bottom to top and all the way to the Gall Bladder, the Liver, the Kidneys, and the Stomach. This set of exercises covers all four of these meridians in a few simple motions.

By massaging the *front* of the legs you are energizing the Liver, Spleen, and Stomach meridians. If you suffer from constant knee joint or back pain, this is also a good place to kick-start the circulation, as it sends vital energy to your muscles and tendons. The *backs* of your legs target the Bladder meridian, and help to ease any discomfort or pain in that organ (see figure 3-18). The *sides* of your legs energize the Gall Bladder meridian, and the *inside* of your thighs is a straight path to the Liver, Spleen, and Kidneys.

Lower Body Patting Exercise

Step One: Remain standing and place both hands on your lower back, patting *down* the *back* of both legs, over the buttocks down to your ankle. Then, place your palms on the front of your ankles and pat *up* the *front* of the leg past

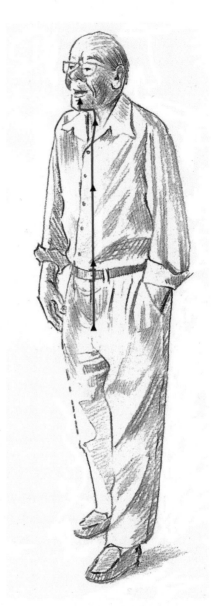

Figure 3-17. Ren Mai or Conception Vessel

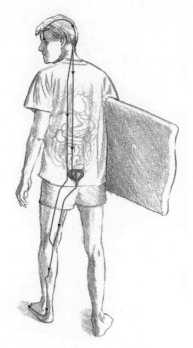

Figure 3-18. The Bladder Meridian

the knees until you reach your waist (see figure 3-19). On the way *down*, you are energizing the Bladder meridian. On the way *up*, you are stimulating the meridians of your Liver, Stomach, and Spleen.

Next, pat your hands down the *side* of your legs to the ankle, then finish by continuing up your *inner thighs*, back to your groin. These four motions, down the back, up the front, down the sides, and up the inner thighs, should be done in rapid succession, in one fluid movement. Make sure to do seven times.

Step Two: Finally, relax and shake out your legs seven times to loosen your hips and relax your shoulders.

Part Six
Creating Energy Through Breath

The Lungs are pretty miraculous mechanisms. They take the invisible air and Qi that you breathe from the outside and transform it into useful energy. This is why the Lungs are considered the Qi leaders of the body, and why creating a healthy airflow to these organs is so vital. A strong, healthy exchange of oxygen is central in keeping your Lung capacity strong and resilient, so that you can withstand physical and emotional attacks. Each and every breath actually boosts the circulation of Qi throughout your body, making a powerful Lung workout essential to total health.

Breathing Exercises

Step One: Start by standing tall, with your feet slightly apart. Take a deep breath and hold it while raising your left arm overhead. Now, exhale through your mouth and slowly drop your hand to your side. Repeat on the right side. Do this exercise a total of five times on each side (see figure 3-20).

Step Two: Once again, raise your left arm straight overhead. Inhale deeply through your nose and place your left hand on the back of your neck. Hold it for four counts. Exhale through your mouth as you drop that arm gently to your side. This opens your chest and expands Lung capacity. Repeat on the right side, for a total of five times on each side (see figure 3-21).

Step Three: Stand up straight with your hands by your sides. Inhale deeply. Hold the breath, then scrunch your shoulder to your ear. After a few seconds, exhale and relax your shoulders. Do this exercise five times on each side.

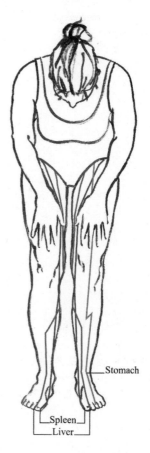

Figure 3-19. Energizing Front Meridians

You have now completed my daily internal organ exercises. Feels better already, right?

Create a Consistent Practice

By learning to cultivate and strengthen Qi throughout your body, you are actively engaged in fortifying its healing ability. It's a lot like

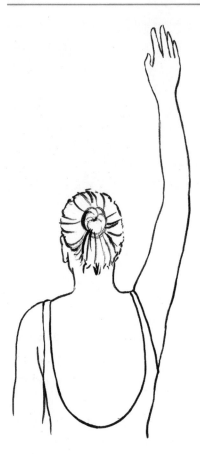

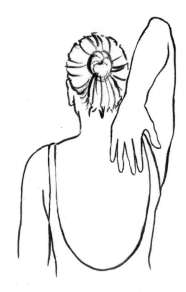

Figure 3-20. Breathing Exercises,
Step One

Figure 3-21. Breathing Exercises,
Step Two

training your muscles for a long-distance marathon. Build slowly, day after day, and your body will gradually make the gains it needs.

Once you feel at home and familiar with these exercises, they are easy to share with your friends and family. Remember, it's easy to adapt these exercises to all age groups. If your spouse or children are reluctant, start by giving them a demonstration. My female patients tell me their husbands have become ardent converts the moment they receive a first-thing-in-the-morning meridian massage.

I personally use these exercises every morning. Before getting out of bed I sit up and massage my hands and feet, then move on to my head, face, and ears. Once I'm standing, I knead the inside and outside of my arms and continue with the rest of the massage sequence.

Since most every living creature has energy meridians, you can also adapt these exercises to the

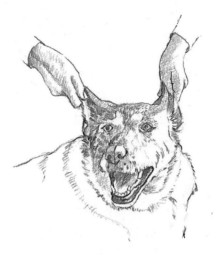

Your pet has meridians, too.

furry friends in your home. They, too, suffer some of the same health problems as humans—lethargy, aggression, overeating. Why not try massaging their energy pathways and see if it improves their behavior?

Before you take your pets for a walk in the morning, tap the insides of their legs to access the Kidneys, Liver, Lungs, Spleen, and Heart. Stroke the outside of their legs to contact the Colon, Small Intestine, Gall Bladder, and Triple Heater. And don't forget your pets' face and ears. The ears contain every acupuncture point for their entire body. Animals love this attention, and will enjoy it as a pre- or postwalk treat. For more information on acupuncture for your pets, check the resources for animal veterinary acupuncture.

The Importance of Touch

Unfortunately, we don't always take the time to give ourselves a gentle massage. It's certainly understandable, but by ignoring this fundamental need, you are denying your physical self. To be truly well balanced, try cultivating the flow of Qi by using these gentle, simple steps. Done properly, the effort expended on the outside of your body will pay off on the inside, keeping your entire energy network healthy over the long haul.

Not only do these exercises feel good, but they also calm and soothe your nervous system. I have personally seen improvements in everything from sinus problems to asthma and chronic fatigue. They also work for patients with heart palpitations, digestive problems, depression, and other serious ailments.

Don't be afraid. Massage those meridians. Breathe deeply. Get out and move. By making a daily commitment to your body, you are taking positive steps to take control of your health. In my experience, there is no greater gift than the healing touch that everyone is capable of providing.

DR. TING'S TOTAL HEALTH ESSENTIALS

ESTHER TING'S MERIDIAN EXERCISE

1. **Hands:** Massage inside, outside of hands (1x each hand). Affects the Heart, Small Intestine, Pericardium, Triple Heater, Lungs, and Colon. Massage the front of the hand, back of the hand, and each of the five fingers, from bottom to top and back again.

2. **Feet:** Massage the soles, top of the feet, and each of the five toes, top to bottom (1x each foot). Affects the Stomach, Spleen, Liver, Gall Bladder, and Kidneys.

3. **Head/Face:** Massage the scalp, eyes, and ears (6x). Affects the Liver, Gall Bladder, Lungs, Colon, Stomach, Kidneys, Bladder, Small Intestine, and Conception and Governing Vessels.

4. **Upper Body:** Pat the arms, inside and outside (7x). Affects the Lungs, Colon, Heart, Pericardium, Triple Heater, and Conception Vessel.

5. **Lower Body:** Pat the legs along the back, front, and sides (7x). Affects the Liver, Gall Bladder, Kidneys, Bladder, Stomach, and Spleen.

6. **Breathing:** Inhale, arms raised (5x). Inhale, arms bent (5x). Affects the Lungs and Colon.

4

Nourish and Fuel
The Healing Power of Food

If there's one thing I can say with total certainty, it's that Chinese people love to eat. When I close my eyes, I can still conjure up the aroma of mung bean soup wafting from our family kitchen on Shanghai's West Nanjing Street, where I grew up.

In China, food is more than simply nutrition; it's also a significant part of daily life.

All around Shanghai and other major cities, you'll find entire city blocks packed with restaurants. Our love of food is even part of the language. *"Ni chi le ma?"* isn't just a common phrase for "hello"; it also means, "Hi, have you eaten?"

We believe that food isn't something that takes up room in your stomach—it actually has the ability to *heal disease*. In fact, Chinese doctors have used this knowledge of food and its healing properties for thousands of years, regularly prescribing specific diets along with their herbal formulas and acupuncture treatments.

Healing with Food: How Much Is Enough?

I grew up during a very difficult economic period in China's history. Throughout World War II, the Great Famine of China, and the Cultural Revolution, food was hard to come by. In those times the government developed a rationing system, and each family was given vouchers for its monthly ration of rice, fish, dairy, and sugar. In my family, all eight of us survived for an entire month on rice, eight ounces of oil, two ounces of sugar, four ounces of meat, and a pound of eggs.

Imagine my astonishment upon arriving in the United States twenty-five years ago. I could not believe my eyes: supermarkets were as big as an entire city block. And the sheer amount of food— such choices! There were countless varieties of everything; even the dairy case had fifty varieties of cheese. And best of all, no lines. To me, this abundance of food was *better* than a fat bank account. I suddenly felt rich beyond my wildest dreams. I would never go hungry again.

But along with this great abundance, comes a Pandora's Box of choices. Despite this tremendous variety and wealth of food, people all over the world are experiencing obesity and disease in epidemic proportions. This is where the Chinese way of eating healthy can make a difference.

In China, we believe that it is possible to enjoy foods of every kind: beef, potatoes, even a piece of cake now and then. The important thing is to understand your body and its particular needs, to choose fresh foods with a strong life force, and to eat in moderation.

People are accustomed to feeding themselves according to what's available at a given moment. They eat what is quick, tasty, and fashionable. But in the process they have lost touch with their bodies and what is good for them.

Healing with Food: Food as Fuel

In the West, food is often evaluated in terms of numbers and percentages. My patients are forever explaining how they count every calorie and measure their carbohydrates and fats. They're usually surprised when I explain that I look at food very differently.

Chinese physicians have used foods to heal the human body for over three thousand years. It all started with a fifteen-hundred-year-old book called *One Thousand Ounces of Gold*. Strange title for a book about food, right? Well, its author, Dr. Sun Szu-miao, believed that the human body was actually more precious than one thousand ounces of gold. That's how vital he felt food was to nourishing and restoring the human body.

Dr. Sun stressed that what you eat is the fuel that makes your body run—which is why choosing and preparing a healthy and balanced meal three times a day is so important. Regular nourishment and nutrition keeps energy flowing freely throughout your various channels and power centers. This even flow of energy is the key to helping you stay healthy and strong. I was recently reminded of this lesson in a very personal way.

Healing with Food: How Powerful Is Your Engine?

One morning a few years ago, I was heading out the door when I got a call from my 104-year-old aunt. Even at this remarkable age she remained astonishingly strong and healthy, living in her own home, eating and walking unattended.

But on this day I could tell from her voice that she wasn't her usual, confident self. When I got her to calm down my aunt told me why she was so upset. She hadn't slept and eaten for two days and couldn't move a muscle. Her joints had literally "locked up." Fortunately, I had a pretty good idea what she was experiencing and told her I'd be right over.

As it happened, it was Mother's Day, and I had already promised to take her out for lunch. Even though she wanted to stay home, I persuaded her to stick to our plans. Normally the first one out the door, this time she needed help. After dressing her, I carried her out to the car, all the while staying bright and positive.

At the restaurant I seated her at the best booth, and immediately ordered a sumptuous dim sum lunch. We laughed and joked, and lo and behold, after a few bites, my aunt began to revive. By the end of the meal, she had eaten twice what I had, and walked out to the car completely unattended, brushing off any attempts to escort her.

How could food have made such a difference?

A good way to visualize this process is to think of a car engine. Food is the "gasoline" or fuel that enters the body in a raw state. The Stomach, Spleen, and Small Intestine filter, separate, and refine that fuel, creating Blood and Qi, the rich nutritious soup that powers the body's organs, nervous system, and brain. But if you run out of this precious fuel, the engine sputters to a stop, and so do you.

In Chinese medicine, rich, protein-laden Blood is a nutritive substance and is fundamental to all facets of your physical and mental health. Qi is the vital spark that makes it all possible. Working jointly, these substances provide the energetic glue that holds you together.

When my aunt told me her joints had locked up, I had my first clue as to what was causing her distress. I knew immediately that there wasn't enough Blood in her system. Because of her advanced age, her Blood and Qi were already flowing at a slower pace. When she stopped eating, it was clear that the vital force that food gave her had literally dried up. To conserve energy, her Heart then reduced the flow of Blood to her five power centers.

Since all five power centers are interrelated, this kind of energy shortage is often connected to other organs—the Kidneys, for instance. Your ministry of power is in charge of supplying an even flow, and this organ system is most easily affected by the emotion of fear. In my aunt's case, a combination of physical and emotional events was responsible for causing her entire body to stiffen. Naturally, she became fatigued and anxious and was unable to sleep. No wonder she called me in a panic.

As soon as she ate her lunch of dim sum, her Kidneys and the rest of her body began receiving the fuel it needed, and kicked into gear. The love and laughter around the table also gave her Heart the energy it needed to pump much-needed Blood to her muscles and tendons.

FOOD FOR THOUGHT

If your children are nodding off at school, and their work is suffering, keep tabs on what they eat. It's important for them to have a solid meal at breakfast, including some protein, such as eggs or milk; even some peanut butter on toast can be beneficial. Without the proper fuel, there is not enough Blood and Qi pumping through the body, and the brain cannot function properly.

Food equals life. It's that simple. This is why eating three meals a day on a regular basis is so vitally important. Each time you skip a meal, you are robbing your human engine of Blood and Qi, the precious fuels needed to keep your engine running.

But just as with an engine in a car, you also have to know what grade of gasoline to put in the tank. And that means knowing more about your body's specifications.

What Kind of Engine Do You Have?

To keep your engine running smoothly, you need to maintain it regularly. If it gets too *hot*, your motor overheats. If the fluids that keep it lubricated run dry, the engine seizes. A winter freeze can cause parts to cool and contract, affecting your ability to lubricate all your vital parts.

Let any of these things happen and the body breaks down. This is when a patient usually decides to see me.

To determine what exactly is going on inside your engine, Chinese medicine differentiates between six temperature and energy patterns: **Hot, Cold, Dry, Damp,** Underpowered, and Overpowered (or as we call it, **Deficient** and **Excessive**). Simply put, these six patterns give us clues to evaluate the present state of your health and wellness.

If you tend to run **Hot**, I usually notice a reddish complexion, hard stools, and scanty urine. Often this comes with an unquenchable thirst for ice-cold drinks.

On the other hand, if you have a pale, whitish complexion and a pale tongue with a thin white coating; suffer from stubborn, runny mucus; and prefer hot or warm drinks, it may mean you are running **Cold.**

If you suffer from itchy, **Dry** skin and rashes, it might often be accompanied with dry mouth, dry eyes, dry cough, or a dry stool.

TABLE 4-1

TEMPERATURE TYPES
Hot
Cold
Dry
Damp

ENERGY TYPES
Excessive
Deficient

Additionally, if you often feel sluggish, heavy, and tired, and your tongue looks **Damp**, glossy, or greasy, you may also suffer from swollen ankles or have difficulty losing weight.

Underpowered (**Deficient**) and overpowered (**Excessive**) patterns have to do with the kind of energy you are projecting. If your engine is weak or underpowered, it stalls and stops moving. Run yourself too hard, and everything can explode.

A person with an **Excessive** constitution is generally someone who is strong, energetic, and easily excited. This person has a reddish complexion can be very combative, self-righteous, and talkative; and may suffer from hypertension.

A person with a **Deficient** physical constitution has low energy and is often depressed. This person might be pale, underweight, or skinny; perspire easily; and suffer from hot flashes as well as shortness of breath.

This is precisely why it's important to know what *kind* of engine you have. Just like that car, it tells you what type of fuel is right for your unique body and energy pattern.

Most people combine a mix of these energy and temperature patterns. You can get a good idea of what kind of body type best describes you by taking the following quiz.

How Hot Does Your Engine Run?

A Quiz to Determine Your Body's Temperature and Energy Level

Put a check next to each statement that accurately describes your present health condition or pattern.

I HAVE:

___ Red eyes (A)

___ Hot flashes (A)

___ Bright red complexion (A)

___ Excessive perspiration (A)

___ Fever (A)

___ Skin eruptions (A)

___ Fainting spells (A)

___ Delirium (A)

___ Disturbed sleep (A)

___ Swollen glands (A)

___ Dark urine (A)

___ Heat rash (A)

___ Swollen joints (A)

___ Craving for cold, icy drinks (A)

I HAVE:

___ Thick mucus in mouth, nose, and throat (B)

___ A tendency to bloat (B)

___ A tendency to gain weight and difficulty with losing weight (B)

___ Feelings of sluggishness and heaviness (B)

___ Digestive issues: indigestion, abdominal pain, excess stomach acid (B)

___ Issues with obesity (B)

___ Anorexia or bulimia (B)

___ Fibroid tumors (B)

___ Hemorrhoids (B)

___ Blood sugar disturbances (B)

___ Craving for sweets (B)

___ Joint pain (B)

___ Varicose veins (B)

I HAVE:

___ Pale, ashen complexion (C)

___ Severe lower back pain (C)

___ Impotence(C)

___ Frigidity (C)

___ Loss of libido (C)

___ Prostate problems (C)

___ Fatigue (C)

___ Loss of endurance (C)

___ Craving for warm drinks (C)

___ Tendency to feel cold(C)

___ Cold extremities: cold hands, cold feet (C)

___ Chronic cold weather illnesses (C)

___ Brittle bones(C)

I HAVE:

___ Dry brittle hair and nails (D)

___ Dry mouth (D)

___ Dry nasal passages and sinuses (D)

___ Dry skin that wrinkles easily (D)

___ Dry irritated skin (D)

___ Dry cough (D)

___ Tightness of chest (D)

___ Constipation (D)

___ Low urine (D)

___ Lack of vaginal lubrication (D)

___ Eczema (D)

___ Psoriasis (D)

___ Dandruff (D)

___ Dry, scaly pimples (D)

I HAVE:

___ Pale, ashen complexion (E)

___ Lack of energy, exhaustion (E)

___ Menstrual irregularities, (missed periods, light or short flows) (E)

___ Shallow breathing (E)

___ Low libido (E)

___ Low blood pressure (E)

___ Lightheadedness, dizziness (E)

___ Low appetite (E)

___ Lack of saliva (E)

___ Weak, poor muscle tone (E)

___ Lack of endurance (E)

___ Depression (E)

___ Depleted, weakened immune function (E)

___ Immune deficient disorders, such as chronic fatigue or lupus (E)

I HAVE:

___ High blood pressure (F)

___ Excessive PMS symptoms, including severe cramping, abdominal distention, severe headaches, severe emotional mood swings, anger, intense irritability, or acute anxiety (F)

___ Excessive perspiration (F)

___ Erratic pulse (F)

___ Excess saliva (F)

___ Heavy menstrual flow (F)

___ Excess appetite (F)

___ Excessive allergic symptoms (F)

___ Acute flare-ups of arthritis (F)

___ Hypersensitivity to light and loud noises (F)

___ Rapid speech (F)

___ Excessive giggling (F)

___ Hysteria (F)

___ Explosive energy (F)

SCORING THE QUESTIONNAIRE

Count up the boxes you've checked in each category and enter the total amount in the chart below.

A	B	C	D	E	F
(HOT)	(DAMP)	(COLD)	(DRY)	(DEFICIENT)	(EXCESSIVE)
___	___	___	___	___	___

These totals are meant as general guidelines that will show you which energy patterns best describe you at this point in time.

You may find that you identify strongly with one particular temperature or pattern. For example, if the D column has more checks than the C column, you are exhibiting more of a dry state than a cold one. Most likely, however, you'll have a mixture of patterns; in other words, you may show a Hot/Dry pattern, or a Deficient/Cold pattern.

This is where Chinese medicine differs from a Western diagnosis. Rather than defining an illness through measurements and numbers, a practitioner will characterize disorders by internal and external causes, as well as by energy and temperature patterns. Again, these are not necessarily permanent categories, but simply a temporary guide to help you pinpoint your current condition. For example, if you are running Dry, you might begin by asking yourself a few questions: Are you living in a dry environment? What kinds of foods are you eating? If you are running Cold and Deficient, have you been exposed to cold weather or cold temperatures recently? Have you been

under a lot of emotional stress or fear? Is there a person or situation
that is "draining" your energy?

Since everyone's engine is different and unique, a Chinese physician can be much more precise about which of these patterns you are
showing. Later chapters will refer back to these energy patterns and
you will be able to explore specific exercises, therapies, and treatments. There are a lot of things you can do on your own, however, to
manage your symptoms.

One of the simplest ways to feel healthier and stronger is to watch
what you eat. The food choices you make can balance these unique
energy and temperature patterns.

Healing with Food: Food and Food Temperatures

Throughout thousands of years of record keeping and meticulous
case studies, the Chinese have paid close attention to food and food
groups and how they affect the human body. Strange as it may
sound, just as the human body can be characterized by different
temperature and energy patterns, food is also classified according its
own unique temperature.

TABLE 4-2. FOOD THERMOMETER

Hot
Warm
Neutral
Cool
Cold

When Chinese physicians talk about the temperature of a given
food, they don't mean, "Does a hot piece of pizza burn your tongue?"

They are referring to whether a particular food *heats* your body or *cools* it down. A chile pepper, for example, is not hot to the touch. But what does your body do when that pepper hits your esophagus? Your mouth begins to sizzle, every pore exploding with spicy fire. That is your body heating up.

The same effect holds true for foods having the opposite temperature. Ice cream is a good example. It might be cold to the touch, but the average scoop is loaded with a processed sugar content that actually produces a *warming* energy in the body. It also has a high dairy content, which increases the levels of mucus and *dampness*.

The temperature of food is determined by the effect it has on the body. Just like the Five Devils discussed in chapter 2, food comes in five distinct temperatures—**Hot, Cold, Warm, Cool,** and **Neutral**.

By looking at the charts on the following pages (see table 4-3, page 100), you can get a good idea of some typical foods and their temperature categories:

Hot and Warming foods: Onions and chicken move energy upward and outward, helping the body to perspire and release toxins locked inside. They also help to smooth the process of circulation and digestion. If you have a cold or flu, for example, I might prescribe warming herbs, as well as recommend a recipe for chicken soup, boiled for an hour with ginger and onions.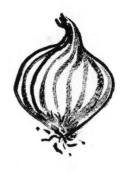

The goal here is to use herbs and food to induce that outward movement of yang energy, and "kick" the virus out of your body.

If you are running Cold, the general rule is to eat more warming foods, such as onions, as well as more protein from other foods like chicken or lamb. Of course, if you suffer from Heat symptoms—a sunburn, for instance—these warming foods would have a negative effect, so something more cooling would be called for.

ESTHER'S WARMING CHICKEN SOUP TO KICK OUT THE FLU

YIELD: 6 TO 8 SERVINGS

INGREDIENTS:
ONE WHOLE YOUNG CHICKEN
3 SMALL PIECES OF GINGER, SLICED THE SIZE OF A QUARTER, 1/4 INCH
THICK
1 LARGE ONION
2 RIBS CELERY, CUT IN HALF
1 BUNCH PARSLEY
1 BUNCH DILL
SALT AND PEPPER

Place the entire chicken and ginger in a large pot. Add water to cover. Boil for 45 minutes. Add the vegetables and simmer for 10 minutes, until soft. Remove the chicken, debone it, and add it to the bowl. Skim off fat from the broth, if any, and season to taste. Add the broth and vegetables to the bowl, inhale the aroma, and enjoy!

It's important to note that not all foods of the same family have the same temperature properties. Take the bean family, for instance. A kidney bean is considered drying, while a soybean has more moistening characteristics (see table 4-3).

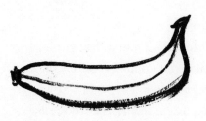

Cold and Cooling foods: Pork, celery, watermelon, or bananas direct energy inward and down, slowing the flow of energy in the body and cooling your upper and outer parts. If you suffer from inflammation and heat, cooling foods such as watermelon, cucumbers, or mung beans are best.

Neutral foods: Beef, carrots, and sweet potatoes tend to balance all conditions. If you're unsure where to start, these foods can be safely added to nearly any diet without ill effects.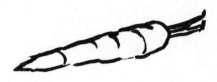

Moistening foods: Pears or honey lubricate your body when you are suffering from dry symptoms such as parched skin or a dry cough.

Drying foods: Kidney beans, celery, and barley drain excess Dampness. If you are overweight, retain a lot of water or are feeling sluggish, it is best to eat things that allow fluids to pass through your body quickly.

Energy foods: Eggs, beef, black beans, almonds, or walnuts strengthen any type of energy deficiency, improving symptoms such as listlessness or fatigue. If your ministry of power is running low, think about eating protein-filled foods such as these to strengthen the Blood.

Calming and clearing foods: Raw vegetables, fruits, and fish reduce excessive energy if you are experiencing symptoms such as hypertension and high blood pressure.

Healing with Food: Mix and Match

How does food help fight disease or illness? All foods have healing properties beyond just their nutritional value. Many of my patients have been able to speed up their healing process just by mixing and matching some of the food groups they eat every day. It's done by carefully watching any untoward symptoms.

TABLE 4-3.
THE TEMPERATURES OF FOOD

HOT FOODS
For Cold Conditions

Black Pepper	Cottonseed	Green Pepper	Soybean Oil
Cinnamon Bark	Ginger (dried)	Red Pepper	White Pepper

WARMING FOODS
For Cold Conditions

Apricot Seed	Coriander	Kumquat	Refined sugar, flour
Brown Sugar	Date (Red, Black)	Lamb	Raspberry
Butter	Dill	Leek	Rosemary
Caraway	Eel	Litchi	Shrimp
Cherry	Fennel	Longan	Spearmint
Chestnut	Garlic	Maltose	Squash
Chicken	Ginger (Fresh)	Mutton	Star Anise
Chive	Ginseng	Mustard Leaf	Sunflower Seed
Cinnamon Twig	Grapefruit Peel	Nutmeg	Sweet Basil
Clove	Green Onion	Onion	Sword Bean
Coconut	Guava	Peach	Vinegar
Coffee	Ham		

COLD FOODS
For Hot/Warm Conditions

Bamboo Shoot	Clam Shell	Lettuce	Sugar Cane
Banana	Crab	Persimmon	Water Chestnut
Clam (salt and	Grapefruit	Salt	Watermelon
fresh water)	Kelp	Seaweed	Yogurt

COOLING FOODS
For Hot/Warm Conditions

Amaranth	Lettuce	Pear	Tofu
Apple	Lily Flower	Peppermint	Tomato
Barley	Mandarin Orange	Rabbit	Wheat
Bean Curd	Mango	Radish	Wheat Bran
Button Mushroom	Marjoram	Sesame Oil	Wheat Germ
Chicken egg white	Millet	Spinach	Wild Rice
Cucumber	Mung Bean	Strawberry	Whole Wheat
Eggplant	Oyster Shell	Tangerine	

CALMING/CLEARING FOODS
For Excessive Conditions

Banana	Clove	Orange Peel	Spearmint
Basil	Corn Oil	Peach	Tangerine Peel
Caraway	Hawthorne Berry	Peanut Oil	Tomato
Carrot	Honey	Persimmon	Turmeric
Celery	Kelp	Seaweed	Vinegar
Clams	Mung Bean	Sesame Oil	

DRYING FOODS
For Damp Conditions

Adzuki Bean	Corn	Horseradish	Parsley
Anchovy	Daikon Radish	Kidney Bean	Pumpkin
Barley	Garlic	Lemon	Radish
Button Mushroom	Green Tea	Marjoram	Scallion
Celery	Jasmine Tea	Mustard Leaf Onion	Turnip

LUBRICATING FOODS
For Drying Conditions

Almonds	Eggs	Peanut	Seaweeds
Apple	Herring	Pear	Sesame Seed
Banana	Honey	Persimmon	Soybeans
Barley	Millet	Pine Nut	Spinach
Clam	Oyster	Pork	Tofu
Dairy			

NEUTRAL FOODS
For All Conditions

Abalone	Corn Silk	Liver (Beef)	Rice Bran
Adzuki Bean	Crab Apple	Liver (Pork)	Salmon
Apricot	Cuttle Fish	Lotus Fruit (Seeds)	Saffron
Beef	Duck	Mackerel	Sardine
Beetroot	Egg	Milk (Cow, Human)	Shiitake mushroom
Black Fungus	Egg yolk	Olive	Sour plum
Black Sesame Seed	Fig	Oyster	Sunflower Seed
Black Soybean	Grape	Papaya	Sweet Rice
Bok Choy	Guava Leaf	Peanut	Sweet Potato
Cabbage (Chinese)	Honey	Pineapple	Taro
Carrot	Herring	Plum	White Fungus
Celery	Kidney Bean	Pork	White Fish
Chicken egg	Kidney (Pork)	Potato	White Rice
Chicken egg yolk	Kohlrabi	Pumpkin	Yam
Corn	Licorice	Radish Leaf	Yellow Soybean

STRENGTHENING FOODS
For Deficient Conditions

Apple	Clam	Kidney Bean	Sardine
Apricot	Dandelion	Lentil	Spinach
Asparagus	Dark Leafy Greens	Liver	String Bean
Beef	Date	Milk	Sweet Rice
Black Sesame Seed	Eel	Oats	Tofu
Bone Marrow	Fig	Oyster	Tomato
Cheese	Ginseng	Parsley	Watercress
Cherry	Grape	Pear	Watermelon
Chicken	Ham	Pork	Yam
Chinese Red Dates	Honey	Potato	

TABLE 4-4. FOOD AND TEMPERATURE GUIDELINES

If you have **Heat** symptoms, such as:

Red, eyes	Delirium
Hot flashes	Disturbed sleep
Bright red complexion	Swollen glands
Excessive perspiration	Dark urine
Fever	Heat rash
Skin eruptions	Swollen joints
Fainting spells	Craving for cold, icy drinks

Limit Hot and Warming foods such as:

Refined white sugar (warming)	Spicy foods and vegetables (curries,
Alcohol (warming)	onions, peppers, garlic)
Caffeine (warming)	Warming grains (oats)
	Warming fatty meats (lamb, beef, chicken)

Enjoy Cooling foods, Neutral foods

If you have **Cold** symptoms such as:

Pale, ashen complexion	Loss of endurance
Severe lower back pain	Craving for warm drinks
Impotence	Tendency to feel cold
Frigidity	Cold extremities: cold hands, cold feet
Loss of libido	Chronic cold weather illnesses
Prostate problems	Brittle bones
Fatigue	

Limit Cold and Cooling foods such as:

Cooling raw vegetables and fruits	Cooling seafood (clam, crab)
(bananas, grapefruits, melons,	Cooling grains (wheat bran, whole wheat)
strawberries, watermelon, cucumbers,	
radishes, spinach)	

Enjoy Warming foods, Neutral foods

If you have **Excessive** symptoms such as:

Excessive perspiration	Acute flare-ups of arthritis
Erratic pulse	Hypersensitivity to light and loud noises
Excess saliva	Rapid speech
Heavy menstrual flow	Excessive giggling
Excess appetite	Hysteria
Excessive allergic symptoms	Explosive energy

Limit draining foods such as:

Caffeine	Tobacco
Alcohol	Raw foods

Enjoy Strengthening foods, Neutral foods

*If you have **Deficient** symptoms such as:*

Pale, ashen complexion
Lack of energy, exhaustion
Menstrual irregularities, (missed periods,
light or short flows)
Shallow breathing
Low libido
Low blood pressure
Lightheadedness, dizziness

Low appetite
Lack of saliva
Weak, poor muscle tone
Lack of endurance
Depression
Depleted, weakened immune function
Immune deficient disorders, such as
chronic fatigue and lupus

***Limit** draining and difficult-to-digest foods:*

Caffeine (warming)
Alcohol (warming)
Tobacco (warming)
Raw foods (energy intensive to digest)
Frozen foods

Fried foods
White flour products (pasta, crackers,
bagels, muffins, toast, breads, cookies,
chips, pastries, piecrust)
Salt (cold)

***Enjoy** Strengthening foods, Neutral foods*

---

*If you have **Damp** symptoms such as:*

Thick mucus in mouth, nose, and throat
A tendency to bloat
A tendency to gain weight and difficulty
with losing weight
Feelings of sluggishness and heaviness
Digestive issues: indigestion, abdominal
pain, excess stomach acid
Issues with obesity

Anorexia or bulimia
Fibroid tumors
Hemorrhoids
Blood sugar disturbances
Craving for sweets
Joint pain
Varicose veins

***Limit** Dampening and oily foods such as:*

Fried foods
Dairy products
Frozen dairy products (ice cream)
Dampening fruits and vegetables
(bananas, cucumbers, olives)

Dampening nuts and grains (peanuts,
wheat)
White flour products (pasta, crackers,
bagels, muffins, toast, breads, cookies,
chips, pastries, piecrust)

***Enjoy** Drying foods, Neutral foods*

Maybe you're suffering from hot flashes and red eyes, you crave cold drinks, for example, or you are showing signs of Heat. Try eliminating coffee, sugar, and spicy foods for a few days, and substitute more Cold or Cooling foods, such as apples or cucumbers. Remember, if you continue to eat only Cold foods after a Heat condition has healed, you might feel tired and chilled. In these cases I recommend neutral foods, and see if things improve.

For dry conditions such as eczema, remove Hot and Drying foods—white sugar, onions, alcohol—from your diet for a few weeks. Instead, substitute foods that moisten or lubricate, such as pears and honey. In the case of Dampness and water retention, you might want to hold off on dairy products for a few days, substituting some of the Drying foods on the list. Remember, it is *always* safe to use neutral food groups as a base for all of your meals, and plan from there.

Healing is a process. Give yourself time to experiment. Feel the effects. And try to have a little patience. Sometimes positive results can take a while. The key is to watch and listen to what your body is telling you.

The following guidelines are designed to work with both the tables and the quiz in the previous section. Match up your energy category with the food choices for your specific health pattern. With a little patience, you can create a variety of healthy *and* tasty meals for almost any condition.

Putting It All Together

This information is a general guideline. It is important to keep in mind that every individual is different and may react in unforeseen ways. For best results you may need to experiment a bit before achieving the right combination of foods. And as you heal further, adjustments in diet are usually necessary. The important thing is to choose proper foods—enjoyable foods that help your body heal.

I've seen it often in my practice: After a bit of trial and error, many of my patients have been able to regain control of their health by using food to strengthen and nourish their body-kingdom. It doesn't take much effort and the results can be nothing short of remarkable.

MARIANNE JAS'S STORY: FOOD AS THE ULTIMATE PRESCRIPTION

From a very young age I ate most every meal according to the sage advice of that well-known guide: the food pyramid. Most people remember seeing it posted at the supermarket or school cafeteria wall: an official-looking chart of recommended dietary intake that began with a base of meat, dairy, and carbohydrates topped by fruits, grains, and green stuff. All the basic blocks for maintaining good health.

Just one problem: If those building blocks were so wonderful, then how did I get so sick?

Esther had a simple answer. It was because my diet was not supporting my deficient energy bank account. As she explained it, my body depended on having the right energy level and that level was intricately connected to the types and temperatures of foods I put into my system.

When I started paying close attention, I noticed that each time I'd have a glass of chilled orange juice or some cold yogurt topped with fruit, it would be followed by cramps, diarrhea, and bloating. It seemed that "cold" foods, whether a healthy snack or sugary treat, would make my system react in the same way.

In fact, I often felt the ill effects of cold food even on warm days when everyone else was roasting. Chilled salad or ice cream blizzard, it didn't really matter. I always had the same unpleasant reaction.

Even more oddly, I actually craved *hot* drinks in the midst of a summer heat wave. My husband used to say I was only happy on a scorching afternoon when sipping a steaming cup of coffee or tea.

It turned out there was a good reason for this. Esther explained that Chinese medicine had a name for my condition, and it was called a Deficiency, in my case a Yin Deficiency. I simply did not have enough Blood and Fluids to perform the tasks that were necessary for digestion or to maintain vital energy circulation throughout my body.

By choosing a supposedly "healthy" diet of cold foods made up of raw veggies and yogurt I was actually contributing to the Deficiency. My body had to use excessive amounts of heat and energy to break down the chilled food, resulting in gas and bloating. That was the reason for the constant chilled feeling and my craving for warm food and drinks.

This Deficiency also affected my interior and exterior temperature controls. Eating a handful of cookies or drinking a glass of beer would usually be followed by a surge of Heat through my face and head. Alcohol in particular, Esther told me, often acts like pure gasoline thrown on a fire. The Heat it generates only makes internal fires all the hotter. And since my body didn't have the reserves to cool everything down, I would react instantaneously with immediate headaches and facial rashes.

First, Esther asked me to steer away from "warming foods" such as caffeine and sugar. Then she made me promise that I wouldn't skip any meals. By forgoing a good breakfast in favor of a sugary latte and a Danish, I was robbing myself of protein-rich foods I needed to build Blood and Qi for the day. Instead of the typical three large meals Westerners take for granted, she advocated consistent, lighter meals spaced throughout the day.

By sticking to smaller portions of "neutral" and "strengthening" foods such as eggs, oatmeal, and protein soups, and by eating smaller portions more frequently throughout the day, I immediately noticed a change. I stopped having migraines, and my stomach settled down.

My typical day now often starts with a high energy breakfast of oatmeal mixed with bee pollen, black sesame seeds, honey or molasses, and a tablespoon of high-protein powder (see recipe, page 108). Midmorning, a snack often consists of an egg, perhaps with some peanut butter and crackers. For lunch, a one-pot casserole dish in a slow cooker works wonders. I follow this up with a few walnuts and half a cup of milk, cocoa, and protein powder in the afternoon. If the hunger pangs continue, it's easy to add some tuna or sardines with crackers.

When early evening rolls around, having a bowl of miso soup and a sandwich or maybe a hot salad gives my digestive organs time to settle down for the night. And if somehow I do get an upset stomach, I'll reach for a dose of Stomach Curing Pills, or Gui Pi Wan (see the herbal products in resources section).

By following these simple guidelines, my late-night headaches disappeared completely, along with the distressing stomach cramps and gas. Each morning I wake up with more energy than ever, focused and ready for a new day, a testament to the Chinese way of eating.

Nice knowing you, food pyramid.

The Art of Eating: Tuning In to Your Eating Environment

Given the stresses of modern-day life, most people don't think twice about eating. Food arrives on the plate, we chew it up, swallow, and get on with the day. But this often disconnected relationship with food can affect our health.

When I ask my patients where and when they eat, a lot of them admit they tend to have meals while watching TV, or in front of the computer. At the same time, they're counting calories and fat, and fretting about the effect it will have on their body.

Fortunately, there is a much better way to look at eating. Food is not something to obsess and worry about. The act of choosing and preparing a meal should be fun, something you might want to share with family and friends. My aunt's story is a good example. Her appetite returned once she was able to relax and laugh with those close to her.

MORNING ENERGY MEGA BOOST

YIELD: 1 SERVING

INGREDIENTS:
1/2 CUP WATER OR MILK
1/4 TO 1/2 CUP REGULAR WHOLE OATS
1 TABLESPOON PROTEIN POWDER
1 TEASPOON WALNUTS
1 TEASPOON BLACK SESAME SEEDS
1/2 TEASPOON BEE POLLEN
1 OR 2 FIGS, CUT INTO THIRDS
2 DRIED APRICOTS, CUT IN HALF
1 OR 2 DATES, CUT IN HALF
1 TEASPOON HONEY OR MOLASSES

Place all the ingredients (except the honey) in a small pot. Soak overnight so that oats are softened. In the morning, simmer for 10 minutes, add the honey, and serve.

To keep your digestive organs relaxed and ready to receive food, it's important that you release any residual stress and tension from your body. Take a little extra time with your meals. Savor the taste of your food, and most of all, have fun while you eat. Here are a few simple guidelines.

Esther's Eating Guidelines

Keep it simple: You don't have to stress out about meal preparation. Cook simple dinners a few nights a week. Healthy takeout or leftovers will save time on busy days. Try a Chinese restaurant in your area, where you can get great lunch deals with large portions, and leftovers to take home. In the following table you'll see some recommendations for a tasty and healthy Chinese meal.

HEALING DISHES AT A CHINESE RESTAURANT

If you choose a Chinese restaurant, you can often find some of the most healing and nutritious, not to mention cheapest, menus around . . . if you choose wisely. Now that you know a little bit about Chinese food therapy, it's easy to pick out a delicious, nutritious meal. Generally, I advise my patients to avoid MSG, limit their portion size, and leave some room for leftovers. Finally, it's best to stay away from heavily fried dishes.

For **colds or flu** eat warming dishes such as:
- Steamed or sliced chicken with ginger and onion
- Chicken with garlic and black bean sauce
- Sizzling shrimp with garlic and black bean sauce
- Hot braised shrimp with fresh ginger, garlic, onion, and spicy tomato sauce
- Stir-fried bok choy and mushrooms

For **Heat symptoms**, such as rashes or fevers, eat cooling dishes such as:
- Seaweed and tender tofu soup
- Fresh tofu soup with pork
- Pork chop with spicy salt
- Steamed, salted fish and pork
- Chinese broccoli with oyster sauce
- Snow peas with water chestnuts
- Sautéed asparagus
- Stir-fried tofu with mushrooms
- Steamed crab

For **low energy**, eat strengthening dishes such as:
- Sliced beef with broccoli
- Sliced beef with asparagus and black bean sauce
- Hotpot of brisket of beef with daikon radish
- Shrimp and asparagus with garlic and black bean sauce
- Chicken with asparagus and black bean sauce
- Hot braised string beans
- Crab with garlic and black bean sauce

- Crab with ginger and green onions
- Roast duck
- Peking duck

If suffering from **health- or weight-related issues,** *limit* fried and greasy dishes, such as:
- Kung Pao chicken, scallops, or shrimp
- General Tso's or sesame chicken
- Sweet-and-sour pork
- Deep-fried squid
- Fried clams
- Tangerine beef

Involve children and family in meal preparation (make it a family event): As my grandchildren are always making clear, kids love to be right in the center of kitchen activity. Find easy ways for them to help with dinner, such as breaking up lettuce for a green salad or putting napkins on the table. Older children can help with shopping and boiling water. Involving them in the process not only makes your job easier, it also helps them have ownership in a delicious meal.

Limit the amounts of foods that you eat: Sometimes it's tempting to eat one giant meal of steak or pork, but I always advise my patients to try to eat "a little bit of everything." If you go out to a restaurant and order a large T-bone steak, divide it into smaller portions and let everyone share a bit of protein. Too much red meat clogs your system and creates excessive mucus and phlegm. Likewise, divide your plate of mashed potatoes and trade for a bit of your neighbor's mixed greens. You can have a taste of everything and all will enjoy a more diverse meal.

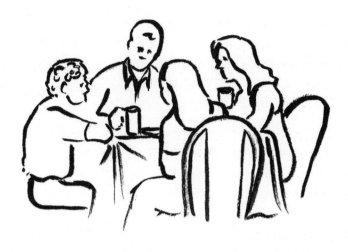

Turn off the television and close that book: It is all too common for people to come home from a long day of concentrating at work, reach for that frozen dinner and quickly eat it, and collapse in front of the TV. Excessive concentration at work or at home affects the ability of the Spleen and Stomach to digest. Instead of continuing to concentrate into the evening, call a friend. Gather the family. Talk with each other. Make eye contact. It's up to you to set the tone!

Chew well: Make it easy for your Spleen and thoroughly chew your food. Not only is it easier to avoid stomachaches but you won't have to expend as much energy digesting.

Limit your intake of cold foods and drinks: When you sit down in a Chinese restaurant the first thing they usually serve is a warm cup of tea. There's a good reason for this. The body uses a lot of energy to warm up cold foods and drinks, so a chronic pattern of Coldness can actually weaken the Spleen's ability to digest. Believe it or not, a small cup of tea or even water at room temperature is all you really need to get your digestive juices moving.

Stop before you're full: Parents often teach us to eat every bite on our plate. That may be a thrifty way to dole out food, but eating too much can cause a road block in your organs and energy channels. If your system is forced to digest excess food that is waiting to be digested, it can make you tired, and cause more work for the Spleen. Overeating puts too much strain on the organs and, over time, can damage your Stomach, Liver, and Heart.

The way to avoid this is to listen to your body. Here's a good rule of thumb: Eat 70 percent of the food on your plate, and leave a few bites. Or better yet, limit the amount of food you put on the plate.

Eat your main meal early: In China we are accustomed to eating the main meal during the middle of the day, rather than later in the evening. This makes sense from a Chinese medical point of view. At night our body and its energy system slows down and gets ready for rest. By forcing it to start the strenuous process of digesting heavy foods a few hours before bed, you are asking it to work overtime. Try smaller, easily digestible meals, such as soups, stews, or broths.

You Are What You Eat

Healing with food does not have to be difficult or expensive. In fact, the best foods are often far cheaper than you might think. And by watching what you eat, you are not only keeping your Wei Qi strong, you're helping to keep illness at bay. Best of all, a delicious meal can actually strengthen your energy pattern.

Food is not just something that takes up space in your stomach—food can heal. Eating the Chinese way is making good foods of every kind work for you. When thinking about what, when, and where you are going to eat, consider your individual temperature and energy level, and try to match it with the temperature and flavor of the right foods that are best for you.

A debilitating flu is a good example. The next time you feel something coming on, boil a few pieces of ginger in a cup of water, or try my recipe for chicken soup. Skip the frozen ice creams and sugary treats until you feel better. By using the simple, fresh foods recommended in the food chart, you will be listening to your body and taking control of your health.

Eat often and in moderation, eat with variety, and above all, relax and have fun. By following the body's unique energy pattern, you can enjoy what you eat without guilt.

DR. TING'S TOTAL HEALTH ESSENTIALS

6 PRIMARY TEMPERATURE/ENERGY PATTERNS

- **Hot:** An increase in body temperature; symptoms can include fever, constipation, skin eruptions, and hypertension.
- **Cold:** A decrease in body temperature accompanied by cold extremities, poor circulation, and pale skin.
- **Dry:** Symptoms include dehydration, extreme thirst, dry skin and hair.
- **Damp:** A moist condition that affects the body with such symptoms as sluggishness and tired, heavy limbs.
- **Excessive:** Too much of something, either Yin, Yang, Heat, Cold, or Fluids.
- **Deficient:** A lack of Blood, Qi, or Fluids within the body, causing an inadequate function of the organs.

5 FOOD TEMPERATURES

- **Hot and Warming foods:** Move energy upward and outward, helping your body to perspire and release toxins locked inside.
- **Cold and Cooling foods**: Slow down the flow of energy in your body and cool your upper and outer parts.
- **Dry Foods:** Drain dampness and fluids.

- **Damp Foods:** Lubricate your body when you are suffering from dry symptoms.
- **Neutral Foods**: Balance all conditions. Can be added to most diets.

FOOD FIXES

- **Heat symptoms:** Limit Hot and Warming foods, enjoy Cooling, Neutral foods.
- **Cold symptoms:** Limit Cold and Cooling foods, enjoy Warming, Neutral foods.
- **Damp symptoms:** Limit Dampening and oily foods, enjoy Drying, Neutral foods.
- **Dry symptoms:** Limit Warming and Drying foods, enjoy Lubricating, Neutral foods.
- **Deficient symptoms:** Limit overly Hot, Cold, as well as hard-to-digest foods, enjoy Strengthening, Neutral foods.
- **Excessive symptoms:** Limit overly Hot or Cold foods as well as Strengthening and Neutral foods.

THE ART OF EATING

- Keep it simple.
- Involve your family.
- Limit your portions.
- Turn off the television/close that book.
- Chew well.
- Limit intake of cold foods and drinks.
- Stop before you're full.
- Eat your main meal early.

5

Relax and Center
Tools for Restoring the Spirit

In this age of sixty-hour workweeks, where days go by in a flash, life can seem more like a game of survival, a gargantuan effort to stay afloat. We rush to appointments. We coach T-ball and soccer. We plan playdates and birthdays. We entertain. We volunteer. We are superhumans.

It's no wonder that a lot of my patients come in complaining of too little time, too little energy, and too many obligations. My first response is always to offer a healing round of acupuncture and herbs. But these are only some of the tools that can be mobilized to calm and heal. To take charge of their health and create a lasting inner peace, I also ask my patients to treat themselves.

This begins by cultivating a spiritual practice that belongs to you, one that calms, soothes, and protects the organs.

Of course everybody has his or her own definition of what it means to be spiritual. You might call it a higher consciousness, or an inner peace. The Chinese have always called it *Shen*.

Just as the Wei Qi protects you against viruses and pathogens, your Shen is your spiritual armor. It calms and soothes your emotions, holding negative influences at bay and keeping your spirit balanced.

Shen is housed in the Heart and, when kept strong, maintains everything from a sense of spirituality to the capacity for love. Alongside those traits are the capability to maintain razor-sharp focus and the determination and wisdom to fulfill your goals. To understand this amazing spiritual force, we need to travel back again in time.

Between Heaven and Earth

The ancient Chinese doctors were healers but they were also philosophers. They came to the conclusion that the healing process works on two levels: the physical, and the spiritual. This was based on a unique idea—that there is Earth and there is Heaven, and we humans take up the space in between. We gain our physical nourishment from the Earth, and receive our spiritual sustenance from the wider universe above. Drawing on each in equal parts provides us with a physical peace that is absolutely vital to a strong Shen. Let them skew out of balance, however, and the Shen becomes disturbed, corrupting decisions and leading to destructive lifestyle habits.

Imagine a beautiful fall day. You're sitting under a tree watching the world go by. Your Qi is flowing and circulating evenly throughout your body. You are relaxed; your Shen, or spirit, is clear and calm. It is in this state that you are best able to make composed and balanced decisions, to glide easily through life's roadblocks. But to reach this restful state you need a strong Shen combined with a vital Wei Qi. Both are essential ingredients for keeping yourself mentally and physically well. It's no surprise, then, that after each diagnosis I often recommend some sort of meditative practice or calming activity. Yes, acupuncture and herbs are fundamental to getting well, but for me, the spiritual part of the healing process is the primary key to curing illness.

Cultivating Shen

My own journey with faith was a bumpy one.

As a young person I had never been particularly spiritual. Apart from some Buddhist ceremonies I sometimes attended at the temple near my home, my family was so focused on day-to-day survival that any spiritual activity was the furthest thing from my mind. Even when the Communist Party came to power and banned *all* religious activity, it had little effect on me.

This changed when I experienced my own brush with death.

As I lay in the cancer ward that dark night in 1979, with severe hemorrhaging and bleeding, I knew how close I was to dying. Here I was, a medical doctor, yet I realized I might never have the chance to accomplish the many things I wanted to do for my family and patients.

Late that night, I felt something give way. I found myself calling out into the darkness, asking the heavens for help. I didn't know if I was being heard, but in the days that followed, I felt an entirely new sensation surging through me.

Gradually, I stopped feeling so alone. I felt calmer, and more certain. My fear and anxiety dried up. And when I went into surgery, I breezed through the operation. A skillful team of doctors removed the cyst, along with my ovaries and uterus. With the help of Western medicine alongside acupuncture and herbs, I healed completely.

My Spiritual Journey

From then on, I began reading spiritual books, Buddhist books, the Bible, books on Chinese Taoism, whatever moved me. And as I did, a strange thing happened. I felt physically better, more calm and less afraid. I also healed faster than anyone anticipated.

How could these spiritual resources have made such a difference? When I went back to my medical texts, I realized the answer was right there in Chinese medicine.

Unlike the Western approach, which teaches that emotions are centered in the brain, Eastern medicine believes that emotions are located in each person's five power centers.

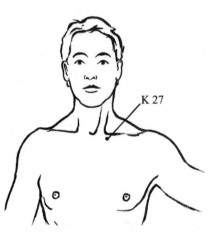

K 27

If you want to release your fear and panic in a stressful situation, press the two points right in the hollow of your collar bone (*Kidney 27*) for a minute or two. Apply firm pressure with the thumb or middle finger. These points are located directly on the Kidney meridian.

Let's look at an example.

Remember the Kidneys and the role they play in transmitting and receiving feelings of fear and panic? As we've seen, those feelings also have a physical effect, one that can cause pain and illness. During that memorable night in the hospital, I had connected with my spiritual self, bonding with a higher consciousness, or Shen. Unwittingly, I was sending calming and soothing signals to my Kidneys, helping them to move my Qi and transition me from a state of fear to a feeling of confidence and peace.

Getting Started

Even if your Chinese physician prescribes herbal and acupuncture treatments, you can further balance your body by using some very simple tools that will keep you peaceful throughout the day.

If you're not sure where to start, try a few different things and see what speaks to you.

It could be a television program, an inspiring book, or maybe a concert with your favorite singer. Some feel that a religious practice works best for them. It could even be something as simple as an inspirational quote or a self-help DVD with meditation techniques. Whatever you choose, it's important to find something that helps keep the world at bay, even if only for a few minutes.

Activating the body's spiritual armor is the best way to protect yourself during stressful times. It doesn't take much to release those emotional pile-ups and send the right energy to your power centers, and it will help you to stay confident and calm.

The following case is a real-life example of the importance of integrating a spiritual practice along with a conventional acupuncture and herbal treatment.

Managing the Pain of Fibromyalgia: Patty

When I first saw Patty, 32, she was emaciated and exhausted. Normally an active, vivacious woman, Patty suffered from involuntary muscle twitches, painful tendons and joints, and severe headaches.

After several of Patty's Western doctors were unable to find any specific symptoms to treat, they finally diagnosed her condition as fibromyalgia, and immediately prescribed beta-blockers to help the pain.

But the medication made it even more difficult for her to function, and Patty's condition worsened. She soon found herself unable to do most everything. Work was impossible; so was driving, even something as simple as writing a check.

I knew exactly how she felt. These were symptoms I had seen many times in other patients both in the United States and China. I had also experienced many of the same things during my own illnesses.

What concerned me most was not Patty's pain or fatigue, but the abnormalities I felt during her pulse diagnosis (see page 248–253). It became clear that, among other things, she was severely Deficient with a lot of Heat in her body, primarily owing to an overactive Liver. This condition had weakened all her other organs as well.

Although Patty's outer demeanor seemed calm and pleasant, her pulse was extremely tight and wiry. This indicated explosive amounts of anger and frustration, emotions that had been in her body for a very long time.

How could I know that?

Using a procedure of examination and diagnosis, I am trained to look inside my patient's power centers, and my diagnosis told me that Patty had kept powerful emotions under wraps since she was a small child.

She admitted that she had suffered abuse, and had since experienced long-term emotional and financial strain. She seemed surprised that this was connected to her present illness. I explained that when these issues are held deep in the organs, they become difficult to release. It can be done, however, and it starts by taking a role in healing yourself.

I put Patty on a program of acupuncture and cooling herbs, and urged her to start cultivating her spiritual side. She began with a

Qigong DVD for beginners, a meditation book and an iPod full of her favorite music. As she got stronger, Patty added some local walks in the mountains. After a few months she was back at work, and feeling much better.

Patty told me that if her experience taught her one lesson, it's that illness is not necessarily a crisis; it also can be a warning signal. When her body finally broke down, it was sending signals that her power centers were overburdened and out of balance.

She discovered, like many of my patients, that calming, centering, and letting go were the keys to maintaining vibrant health.

This is why I always stress the importance of forgiving the past and moving through your traumas. It could be meditation, prayer, or walks in the woods, but whatever you choose, make that connection between your emotions and staying well.

The Healing Power of Nature

Although there are many easy and inexpensive ways to access one's inner strength, nothing touches all of your senses at the same time more than submerging yourself in nature. In the past few years, I have run across many studies emphasizing the benefits of spending more time outside in the natural world. In fact, many corporations are now scheduling "green" retreats for their employees, while schools and hospitals are creating more eco-friendly environments and spaces for learning and healing.

I believe this newfound interest in the natural world is wonderful, and emphasizes something the Chinese physicians have known for centuries: Nature is easily accessible, and touches each of your power centers in a very deep way.

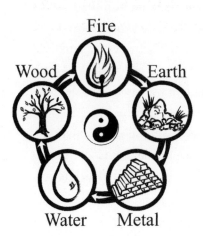

Fire

Wood   Earth

Water   Metal

Figure 5-1. Five Element Sheng Cycle

The Five Elements

Thousands of years ago, the Chinese began closely observing their surroundings. They came to the realization that everything in the universe, no matter how large or small, was made up of one or more of five natural elements: Water, Wood, Fire, Metal, and Earth.

They called their breakthrough the *Wu Hsing*, or Five Element theory, and even today, it forms the very foundation of Chinese medicine. The Five Element theory tells us that not only are plants, oceans, and mountains all made up of these basic elements, but animals and humans also share the same building blocks. They are there within all of us, intricately connected and striving for a proper balance within our body-kingdom. The relationship between these elements is best understood by looking at two distinct cycles: the Creation, or *Sheng*, Cycle (see figure 5-1), and the Control, or *Ke*, Cycle. The Creation cycle works like this:

- **Fire** is the mother of **Earth**.
- **Earth** is the mother of **Metal**.
- **Metal** is the mother of **Water**.
- **Water** is the mother of **Wood**.
- **Wood** is the mother of **Fire**.

The Creation cycle is often called the Mother/Child cycle. This is because the "Mother" element supports the birth and development of the "Child" element that it created. It works like this: When **Fire** burns, the resulting ash creates the **Earth** or soil. When **Earth** weathers and decays, it reveals deposits of **Metal**. These **Metal** and mineral deposits revitalize Water through oceans and riverbeds. **Water** then nourishes the crops and fosters the growth of **Wood**, which encompasses plants, shrubs, and trees. **Wood** gives birth to **Fire,** thus completing the cycle.

The second cycle, called the Control, or *Ke* Cycle, acts as a controlling process, providing checks and balances from element to element. In this cycle, the relationships work almost like a game of rock, paper, scissors:

- **Fire** controls **Metal** by burning and melting it
- **Earth** controls **Water** by damming and absorbing it.
- **Metal** controls **Wood** by cutting it.
- **Water** controls **Fire** by quenching it.
- **Wood** controls **Earth** by way of roots that hold it in place.

Making it a bit more intricate, each one of the elements has a corresponding *organ* within the body; for example, Heart with Fire, Kidneys with Water, and so on (see table 5-1). For the Chinese physician, the interrelationships of these cycles provide an important way to gain insights into a patient's health.

TABLE 5-1

POWER CENTER	RELATED ELEMENT
Heart	Fire
Spleen	Earth
Lungs	Metal
Kidney	Water
Liver	Wood

Treatment Using the Five Elements

This connection between "organs" and "elements" affects the body in very specific ways. Any disruption, and there is a domino-like effect that travels throughout the body. If the Lung becomes weak, it can affect its mother, the Spleen, or its child, the Kidney; even the Liver, the organ it controls. If the Heart becomes weak, it can affect its mother, the Liver; its child, the Spleen; and so on. Once the ancients realized this, they used the Five Element theory to diagnose and treat imbalances just about anywhere in the body.

For example, in the case of insomnia, as a Chinese doctor, I might check to see if your Wood element or Liver is overactive and therefore too dry. From a Five Element perspective, this "burning" Wood (the Liver) could be creating too much fuel, raising the heat and disrupting the Heart (see figure 5-1). Since your Heart houses consciousness, this imbalance might be experienced with feelings of disorientation and agitated nerves. One of the most common treatments would be to cool the Liver/Fire by means of its mother, the Kidney/Water element (see figure 5-1). This is typically done by stimulating unique acupoints that activate these organs, then following up with specially formulated herbal teas or powders.

Another condition I often see is indigestion. Like a root-bound plant, the Liver and its associated Wood element can overpower the Earth element (the Spleen). In this condition, you are unable to receive the nourishment that you need. If you are under a lot of stress, the "roots" of the Wood element soon grow even stronger, taking over and suppressing your appetite. By utilizing Five Element theory, a Chinese physician can prevent further symptoms by calming and releasing the Liver, freeing the Spleen to do its work.

Connecting to the Elements in Nature

The Wu Hsing theory can sound complex, but there are many easy ways to apply it in your own life. First, remember that every person is made up of the five elements, and that each element has a job—to send a healing vibration to its companion power center.

Consider the sensation of a warm campfire on your hands, or the damp Earth between your toes. These natural sensations actually transmit energy, or Qi, to your five power centers, using meridians that begin in your fingers and toes.

The same effect holds true for just about any form of contact with the natural world. This might be an invigorating splash of lake Water or perhaps lying on a mountain slope made up of Earth, minerals, and Metals. These sensations will be picked up by your inner energy receivers and added to the Qi circulating through your energy highways.

This is why each and every one of us needs so badly to be a part of nature. By absorbing Fire, Water, Metal, Earth, and Wood, you actually strengthen and heal your energy circuits, the very life force necessary to stay healthy.

Let's take a closer look at how each of the five elements can calm, restore, and rebuild your energy network.

Fire

The most primal of elements, Fire represents light in the darkness. It warms you when you're cold, and radiates vital energy when you're exhausted. Just as the sun gives life to the earth, the *Fire* element casts its glow on the king of your castle, the Heart.

Fire Element

Who hasn't sat in the sun and felt a sense of joy, or spent a contented evening beside a roaring fire? These aren't just idle sensations. It's the Fire element soothing the Heart and its meridians, and giving it vital energy to stay strong.

By taking advantage of certain times of year when the sun and the Fire element are most prevalent, you can make the most out of their healing properties.

The summer season, for instance, is the time when the Fire element is at its peak. It's a perfect time to organize a barbecue or sit around a campfire with friends or family. Fire's soothing Heat and the intimate connection to family not only strengthens your Fire element, but sends important energy to your Heart and its meridians.

It may seem trivial, but lately science is beginning to see that there is something to this. You may have heard of a condition called SAD (seasonal affective disorder). This is a form of depression caused by lack of exposure to sunlight. It's a good example of how Western medicine has given a name to something Chinese medicine has recognized for thousands of years, and it shows what happens when the Fire element becomes unbalanced.

Keeping conditions such as SAD at bay doesn't have to be difficult. By staying connected to your power centers' need for Fire, you can keep them balanced and working properly. During the winter months, when SAD diagnoses are at their peak, I often recommend some Fire element therapy—simple things like spending some time outside in the sun (fifteen minutes will do), or reading a good book beside a roaring fire.

You can also do some things to bring the Fire element into your home and office. Although these are not an exact substitute for a roaring fire, light a single candle instead, or give the ancient art of Feng Shui a try.

The Healing Art of Feng Shui

Feng Shui (pronounced "fung shway") is the ancient Chinese science of designing living and working structures and placing objects within them for the most beneficial effect. Its name is translated to "Wind and Water," with roots going back to 3000 BC, making it one of the oldest human practices surviving to modern times.

The overall Qi in a home or property can either be harmonious and unified, or it can be tumultuous and filled with conflict. By using Feng Shui to properly arrange the five elements within one's living and working environment, you are actually creating an optimal flow of Qi.

The ideal Feng Shui house is one where all interior objects, colors, and structural design are in perfect harmony with one another and their environment. In many cases, this is done through the help of a Feng Shui expert, who uses tools and formulas based on the solar calendar and the cycles of the seasons to determine a property's unique energy blueprint. You can also try it yourself using various published and online guides; however, the results are usually a bit more hit-and-miss.

Simple things such as clearing your clutter and cleaning the windows, for example, are easy ways keep the Qi in your home flowing smoothly. It is said that keeping the toilet lid closed when not in use prohibits money energy from draining away. Other techniques, such as placing specific colors and elements (water or crystals) in appropriate corners have been known to have good results.

For a local Feng Shui practitioner in your area, try searching online or check the national organizations in our resource section.

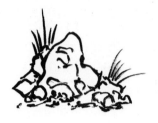

Earth Element

Earth

Have you ever taken a long walk on the beach? Plopped down on a smooth rock? Or plunged your hands into the soil while potting a plant?

All of these sensations give you a warm and healthy feeling, and for good reason: because they connect your body's energy directly with the Earth's. By touching the ground you are contacting the meridians of your Stomach and Spleen, those that are most sensitive to the Earth element.

Your big toe is a good example. The very tip of this toe marks the beginning of your Stomach meridian (see figure 3-10 on page 70). When you step in mud or run along the beach, you are sending Qi through these meridians, directly to your Stomach and digestive organs, strengthening them while you walk.

It's no surprise, then, that if you were to walk through any Chinese city in the early morning, you'll find people doing their early morning Qigong and Tai Chi exercises in the city parks (see pages 140–142 for more about Qigong). These exercises focus on keeping the feet firmly planted on the ground, while the body and arms move in a sequence of poses. And they are a great way to connect to the Earth's Qi. They also help calm the emotions of worry and anxiety, which are connected to the Stomach and Spleen (see box on page 142). An excellent alternative are my internal organ exercises or some earth-centered yoga poses.

YOGA: THE MOUNTAIN POSE

Beneficial for connecting to the Earth's rhythms

STEP ONE

Stand with your feet shoulder-width apart, distributing your body weight equally across your feet.

STEP TWO

Place your arms along your sides and let them hang next to your hips. Remember to inhale and exhale while doing this position.

STEP THREE

Keep your spine aligned and feel it lengthening from the ceiling toward the floor. Keep your head and neck lifted; look forward. Push your legs to the floor and tighten your thighs.

STEP FOUR

Inhale and exhale for a few breaths and continue with your practice session.

Just as Fire has its own season connected to it, so does the Earth. Late summer is a wonderful time to plan some walks or hikes before the colder weather, or to attend an outdoor yoga class or retreat.

Metal

Standing in front of a bronze sculpture or a skyscraper, it's easy to feel a sense of enduring strength. On a smaller scale, consider a solid gold bracelet or an iron fire poker. These metal objects can seem as if they will last forever.

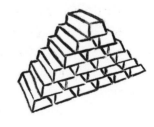

Metal Element

Metal is an element that not only represents the endurance of such materials as copper, silver, and steel, but the richness of gold. It makes sense then that the power center most strengthened by the Metal Element is your body's own structural center, the Lungs.

During Sunday hikes in the local mountains, I often stop on a peak and do a sequence of my breathing exercises. Since autumn is the season for the Metal Element, taking a walk through the fall colors, or even raking some leaves, can do wonders for your Lung energy.

Water

You drink it, you bathe in it, it makes up 90 percent of your body—water is the one element you can't live without. But when it freezes, it becomes hard and unyielding; when it heats, it can evaporate. It's only natural then that the same effects would be true for the water and other fluids in your body.

Water calms and soothes the Kidney energy network.

The organs in charge of distributing water are your Kidneys and Bladder. As you know, their meridians extend from head to foot. By allowing the Water element to touch these meridians, you are directly affecting the body's water department. That's why you need all your fluids to flow smoothly and at an even temperature to maintain your body's systems.

To the Chinese, Water is also a source of unstoppable strength. If you think about a raging river powering through a steep canyon, it's a very powerful image. But Water is also a useful healing tool. When my patients ask me how to stay calm and balanced in their everyday lives, I often advise them to spend some time near a lake or to go swimming in the ocean. Raft a river or just run through the sprinkler

with your kids. The rhythmic pounding of ocean waves or the cool drops
from a hose can do wonders to douse
heated emotions and cool daily stress.

If you don't have a Water source
nearby, invest in a small tabletop waterfall, or a fountain. Even some soothing
Water sounds on a CD can be helpful
in creating the right environment.

Water has a season as well, and
that is winter. It's the time of year associated with frozen Water, which
makes skiing, skating, and snow-
boarding all excellent activities to
stimulate and energize your Kidneys
and Bladder. In fact, a winter outing

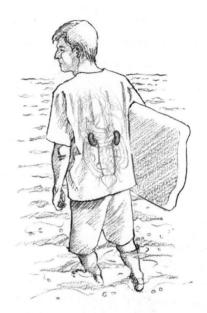

The Water element soothes the Liver
and strengthens the Kidney network.

benefits all five of your power centers.
The mountains and rocks provide the Metal and Earth elements.
The sun reflects the fire element, while plants and trees give you the
Wood element. In reality, just about any outdoor winter activity can
create a whole body experience that touches every part of your
body-kingdom.

Wood

Take a look at a mighty sequoia tree and it's
amazing to think that once a tiny sapling
pushed through the ground to become a tow-
ering, ten-story life force. That is the same
power your Liver holds and why it is connected to the Wood element.

Wood Element

It's not hard to make this connection for yourself. Simply take a leisurely walk or a brisk hike through a forest or park. Your Liver meridians extend all the way to your feet (see figure 3-6 on page 66), so take off your shoes and walk barefoot through the grass. The sensation you feel is the Wood energy surging through your Liver and Gall Bladder channels. It's very much the same energy a plant uses as it stretches out of the ground.

But you don't have to visit a national park to connect to your Liver. Even simple activities such as planting and gardening send vibrations to your Liver's energy circuits.

Notice how every year spring rolls around and you receive those familiar feelings of new growth and possibilities? That's because it's the season associated with the Wood element. During spring, make an extra effort to enjoy fresh plants and flowers. Take the time to see a botanical display, run through the woods, or visit a garden. Any way you can connect to the Wood element pays dividends to your Liver.

The following story is a perfect case in point.

A Half Century in Nature: Paul and Margaret

Paul and Margaret have come a long way since they left their native country of the Netherlands for the United States. They arrived in America just as I did, after surviving a traumatic childhood amid war and famine. Between the two of them they have overcome cancer, heart and intestinal surgery, as well as deep-vein thrombosis.

Yet today, at eighty-plus years old, they are bursting with energy. Both are actively involved in the community. They travel the world, and often take care of their grandchildren for weeks at a time. They even have a daily 5:00 a.m. exercise routine consisting of walks and light weightlifting.

ORGAN	ELEMENT	SEASON
TABLE 5-2		
Heart	Fire	Summer
Spleen	Earth	Late Summer
Lungs	Metal	Autumn
Kidney	Water	Winter
Liver	Wood	Spring

But they have another secret weapon that has kept their immune system able to withstand past traumas and life illnesses.

Every summer for the last forty-five years, they leave their comfortable home to spend a few months camping amid the forests and ponds on Cape Cod.

"Nature revives us," says Margaret. "We couldn't imagine life without it."

For almost half a century they have spent several months a year swimming (Water element), hiking (Wood, Earth, and Metal elements), and of course taking in a crackling campfire (see table 5-2).

"Although we love our home, it's just not the same as eating and sleeping outside," Margaret admits. "Every summer we give the house keys to family and friends and head to a campground nearby."

Without even realizing it, they have been giving their power centers exactly what they need, provided by the natural world, free of charge. In a very real way, they have set their body clocks to nature's own rhythms.

This is exactly what Chinese doctors have been prescribing for centuries. I often ask a patient to visit nature on a regular basis, tailored, of course, to his or her needs. If a person is showing too much Fire, or Heat in the body, I recommend time near the Water. If the Wood or Liver energy is weak, a walk in the forest or a nearby park will do wonders.

Following Paul and Margaret's example is an excellent way to stay healthy and strong. Get outside. Make it a regular habit. Take a swim. Hug a tree. Ride a bike. It's not just good for your muscles; it feeds the very power centers that are vital to a long and happy life.

The Five Colors: The Art of Visualization

As revitalizing as it is to spend time in the outdoors, it's sometimes difficult to find an opportunity in the midst of a hectic day. Fortunately, there are other ways to get some of the same healing benefits, and it's done by using a simple technique called *visualization.*

Visualization is a way of picturing something and imprinting it on your mind before it ever actually happens. It's a technique that has been used successfully by professional athletes in a variety of sports. Tiger Woods, Michael Jordan, and Wayne Gretzky all have used visualization to picture winning their games.

It's not a new technique. Chinese medicine has recommended this practice throughout the ages. It's part of the ancient meditative practice of Qigong, and it's also in Tai Chi, which uses visualization in each and every exercise sequence.

In the last few years Western medical facilities have also used it to reduce anxiety and promote healing in hospital environments. Visualization has even been effective in treating learning difficulties, as well as to increase performance in the workplace.

In Chinese medicine, however, there is a specific technique that focuses on visualizing color. Why color?

Just as there are five elements and five power centers, the Five Element theory teaches that there are also five key *colors* that are instrumental in healing—**red, yellow, white, blue-black,** and **green.** Each color is connected to a specific power center. Red relates to the Heart, yellow to the Stomach and Spleen, white to the Lungs, green to the Liver, and blue/black to the Kidneys.

FIVE ORGANS/FIVE COLORS

Red is the color of your Heart.
Yellow is the color of your Stomach and Spleen.
White is the color of your Lungs.
Green is the color of your Liver.
Blue-black is the color of your Kidneys.

After much study, the ancients found that there is actually a connection between these colors and the way your body interprets them. Today we would call it *color therapy*.

Color therapy has been used far back into human history. Ancient Egypt and India are two of the many cultures that included it in their healing practices. Dr. Sun Szu-miao, a well-known Chinese medical practitioner during the Tang Dynasty, created the first multicolor charts of our meridians and acupressure points

As you will see in chapter 8, a Chinese doctor must be well trained in the use of the five colors. This is because they are the primary tools used in assessing facial color and skin tone during the first stage of diagnosis.

To understand how, think of color and light working in the same way as a sound wave, with each color vibrating at a different rate and frequency. Just as your ears receive high- and low-pitched sounds, the retinas in your eyes also receive light frequencies. These are picked up through blue, green, and red photo receptors called cones.

Color frequencies are also received by your five power centers. This is why, when illness disturbs a particular organ, connecting that organ with the vibration and the energy of its related color can often restore harmony.

The following set of simple visualization exercises is based on an ancient Qigong meditation practice. It uses the five primary colors to calm, soothe, and strengthen your five power centers.

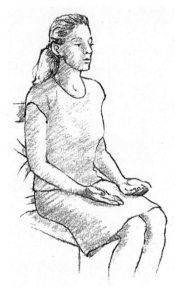

A Meditative Pose

A Color Meditation for Your Five Power Centers

Find a quiet spot, either a chair, a park bench, or even the ground. Sit upright and relax your arms.

You can rest your hands on your knees, palms facing up, or you can clasp both hands in your lap, with the back of the right hand resting lightly on the palm of your left hand. If you already follow a meditation practice, sit in the position that you feel most comfortable with.

Now you are ready to begin.

Red

Red is everywhere—in rocks, in flowers, in the sunset at the end of the day. The color red is the color of the Heart, and the Heart is the primary home for the Shen, or spiritual armor. To keep the Heart and Shen functioning properly, you need to circulate Blood at an even pace.

That is why red is an important color when using visualization.

By sitting quietly and visualizing this color, you will create a vibrational frequency that strengthens the Heart as well as the meridians of its related organs, the Small Intestine, Triple Heater, and Pericardium.

Start by focusing on your Heart area. See it glowing a healthy red. As you're doing this think about a person, place, or experience when you felt joy, happiness, or love. Remember the experience and then smile at the memory. The act of laughing or smiling actually creates

Qi and helps to circulate Blood around your body. Do this every day for the length of ten slow, deep breaths (this will take about two minutes in all).

Each time you activate the color red, you are helping the Heart to keep your Qi moving and flowing throughout the body-kingdom, an important and beneficial addition to your well-being.

Yellow

Yellow might seem like an odd color to be associated with calming and centering, but that's exactly what it does for your Stomach and Spleen meridians. As you've seen, it is the Stomach that extracts and provides nutrients for your body and controls the emotions of anxiety and worry.

If the Stomach becomes dysfunctional, it's usually because you've allowed anxiety to build up. Whether it's a bad day at work, a difficult teenager, or the family finances, when you constantly churn things over and over, your digestive organs start to feel the effects. Foods and fluids aren't put to proper use, nutrients stop breaking down and a feeling of emptiness starts to take over. That, of course, just makes you want to fill up with more foods and fluids, none of which can be broken down efficiently. Eventually, your energy spirals down, along with your ability to think clearly and be productive.

You can head this off, however, by focusing on these organs and visualizing the color yellow.

Close your eyes and picture a deep yellow circle of light. You may want to bask in a soft yellow glow or, if you prefer slightly more healing power, think of the sun and its powerful golden rays. Let this yellow glow radiate from your solar plexus filling your Stomach and digestive organs. Continue this for ten breaths each day.

White

When one sees a bride walking up the aisle in her wedding dress, or a white dove landing in the park, it's easy to conjure up feelings of purity, peace, and innocence. But white is also considered one of the most powerful colors because it includes *all* of the colors in the spectrum. Chinese medicine recognizes this unique fact and endows white with another property: a vibrational frequency that helps to calm and strengthen the Lungs and Colon.

As you may recall, these two organs regulate breathing and waste removal, at the same time as they control emotions of grief and sadness—all reasons to keep your Lungs healthy.

To keep these organs healthy, try visualizing the whitest white light and picture it flowing through every fiber of your Lungs. Breathe deeply and let your feelings release on the out breath. Do this for ten breaths each day.

Keeping your Lung and Colon energy channels moving and flowing gives your entire immune system a better chance of remaining healthy and strong.

Deep Blue-Black

Normally we don't think of black and blue as being one color, but in Chinese medicine they have the same effect on your body. Think about the power and grandeur of the rich blue and black hues of the night sky. By visualizing these colors you are tapping into frequencies that calm and strengthen the Kidney and Bladder. And since both of these power centers store and balance the emotion of fear, we directly affect this critical balance whenever we stop to visualize blue-black.

Start by taking a deep breath, then send a blast of pure, dark blue light to your Kidneys. These two bean-shaped organs are located in your lower back near the pelvic area. Next, imagine this blue light filling up the Bladder and its associated organs. Since the Bladder's meridian runs along the spine, try sending some blue light to that area as well. If you are experiencing pain in your lower back, you'll find this to be a soothing visualization. Do this for ten breaths each day.

Keeping your Kidneys and ministry of power strong is an excellent way to maximize your overall energy supply, as well as keeping the emotion of fear at bay.

Green

Spend any amount of time in nature, and you can't help but notice the color green. In a forest, a garden, or even a potted plant, green is the color of growth. In Chinese medicine it can also be a powerful healing agent that strengthens the Liver and Gall Bladder.

These two power centers are in charge of your ability to plan and strategize. If you feel fragmented or are lacking a cohesive direction, this is a good time to visualize the color green.

Remember, the Liver is the commander, in charge of sending an even flow of Blood and Qi. It is also the organ that controls your feelings of anger and frustration. When it gets stressed, the flow of Blood becomes uneven and choppy, causing symptoms such as heart palpitations and migraine headaches. By resting quietly and picturing a vivid green hue, you are restoring the rhythmic flow of Blood and energy.

The Liver runs the entire length of your ribcage, directly underneath your sternum. Send a blast of green to this area and to your

Gall Bladder, which is nestled below your right rib cage. Do this for ten breaths per day.

Other Calming and Soothing Techniques

Long ago Chinese medicine recognized that when Qi is activated, it loosens up both emotional and physical blockages. Connecting to nature and the Five elements on a daily basis, achieves exactly that. By visualizing and sending the vibration of color to specific areas within the body, we are healing and soothing the organs and their related meridians (see table 5-3).

TABLE 5-3			
ORGAN	ELEMENT	SEASON	COLOR
Heart	Fire	Summer	Red
Spleen	Earth	Late Summer	Yellow
Lungs	Metal	Autumn	White
Kidney	Water	Winter	Blue
Liver	Wood	Spring	Green

As you can see, these therapies are simple, and they have lasting benefits when done on a regular basis. Your body gets the positive Qi it needs to stay balanced, whatever comes your way.

Several other effective practices based on ancient Chinese meditative principles deserve mention. They might seem exotic at first, but again, they are easy to perform and also have long-lasting benefits.

Qigong

Qigong is a series of slow-moving, graceful exercises that combine meditation, breathing, and visualization. The goal is to protect, preserve, and energize the body's Qi as well as strengthen and circulate the Blood. This is done by standing still and focusing on a particular point in the center of the body called the *Dan Tian*, or vital center. This spot is located roughly two inches below the navel and three inches inward (see figure 5-2).

Qigong can be translated as "the principle of cultivating energy." It's not surprising then, that many of China's great scholars and monks such as Confucius and Lao-tzu were Qigong practitioners. They understood that managing and maintaining a rhythmic flow of Qi was essential to our health and vitality.

Across China and in many parts of the world, you can see people of all ages out in the fresh morning air going through their daily Qigong movements. This outdoor ritual is an excellent way to further the connection between the body's five power centers. Many traditional Chinese medical hospitals have even devoted an entire department to medical Qigong, which is used to treat serious illnesses such cancer, brain damage, and stroke. Qigong has also been used successfully in managing and treating a wide variety of immune related disorders, including cancer, fibromyalgia, and AIDS.

Another beneficial exercise is Tai Chi, a close relative to Qigong. Unlike Qigong, which uses movements that come from a still and centered place, Tai Chi is often called "moving in motion." Originating

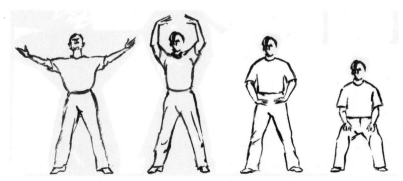

Figure 5-2. Qigong Sequence

from the ancient Chinese martial arts tradition, Tai Chi sequences tend to be longer than those of Qigong, and more movement oriented. If done properly, Tai Chi has tremendous health benefits and is quite beautiful to watch.

If you are interested in learning these ancient practices, I recommend starting with one-on-one instruction, a DVD, or a practitioner in your area; or check the resources section for more details.

BASIC QIGONG SEQUENCE

1. Take a standing position, feet shoulder-width apart, knees relaxed.
2. Turn palms up, spread your fingers apart, and stretch arms to the sides, head held high.
3. Continue bringing hands up; once they are above the head, start exhaling and turn palms down to face the top of the head.
4. Send energy from the center of the palms into the crown of the head.
5. Bring the hands closer to each other as they glide down along the midline of the body. At hip level, palms face down.
6. Repeat steps 2 through 4 several times.
7. Take your seat. Relax. Breathe. Think of nothing. Allow the Qi to circulate and enjoy the feeling of well-being.

Emotional Freedom Technique

Throughout this book I have stressed the connection between emotion and illness. This has always been a fundamental principle of Chinese medicine, but lately it has also attracted the attention of Western clinicians.

Among the techniques they have developed is one particularly effective practice called emotional freedom technique, or EFT. Based on the principles of acupuncture, EFT uses ancient Chinese meridian theory to first identify and then release emotional blockages from the body's power centers. Many people have had extraordinary results with EFT, especially in the area of pain relief, substance abuse, and physical or emotional trauma.

By using many principles of Chinese medicine, EFT has been successful in treating ailments as diverse as fibromyalgia, addiction, weight loss, allergies, phobias, headaches, and ADD/ADHD.

The technique has it roots in the early '80s, with the work of Australian psychologist John Diamond and American psychologist Roger Callahan. Both became intrigued after applying pressure to specific Chinese acupressure points and getting positive results.

In one landmark case, a patient of Dr. Callahan's was able to overcome her lifelong phobia of water by tapping a point on the Stomach meridian directly underneath her eye. Not only did it instantly release her fear, but it also stopped the severe stomach cramps she was experiencing at the time.

This case demonstrates what the Chinese have known for thousands of years: that by pressing or needling these physical or emotional blockages along the body's energy highways, the Qi is freed up, and the problem is corrected.

Drs. Callahan and Diamond continued their research and found that when patients tapped these points while talking through a particular psychological fear or emotional problem, the patients' issues were often resolved more quickly.

In later years Callahan's efforts were further expanded on by Gary Craig, who used it to successfully treat the pain and trauma brought home by Vietnam War veterans. For many, this was the first relief they'd felt in decades.

How does this technique work? It begins with focusing on a specific mental or physical problem while gently tapping eight specific points located on the meridians of the hands and face.

The sequence starts with the meridians of the Bladder, Gall Bladder, Stomach, and Governing and Conception Vessels. We then move on to three more points on the upper torso: the Kidney, Spleen, and Liver (see figure 5-4).

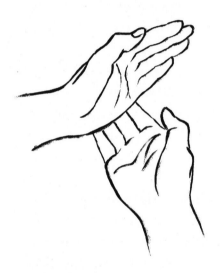

EFT Meridian Sequence

By touching or tapping these points while simultaneously thinking or stating out loud a specific issue or illness, you can actually reverse or unblock an energy traffic jam. Think of it as acupuncture without the needles: It's a cost-free way to remove blockages caused by emotions and pain.

Try the sequence as follows:

1. Think, write, or state the emotional or physical issue that is bothering you. As an example, let's use *my migraine.*

Figure 5-3. Start the EFT sequence by tapping the Karate Chop Point on the Small Intestine meridian.

2. Rate the intensity of the pain or the problem from 0 to 10; 0 is no intensity at all, and 10 is the worst you could feel.

3. Using the second and third fingers of your right hand, lightly tap the point an inch below your pinkie on the fleshy outside part of your palm (see figure 5-3). This point lies on the Small Intestine meridian, and is related to the Heart, the center of your Shen. From

a Chinese perspective, tapping this point awakes the Heart energy and jump-starts the healing.

4. Now state the problem with the desired resolution. *Even though I have this migraine, I'm okay, and I choose to release it now.* Other variations could be : *I accept myself, I love myself, I'm taking care of myself, and I choose to release it now.*

5. After tapping the side of your hand, and repeating the problem and resolution three times, narrow your words down to *this migraine*, or *this problem*, and you're ready to start the sequence.

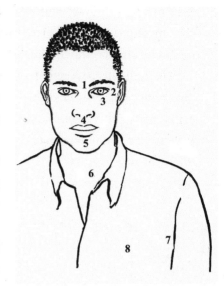

Figure 5-4. EFT Meridian Sequence

6. Next, with the same two fingers on your right hand, start tapping the eight-point acupressure sequence (see figure 5-4). Tap the inner eyebrow (#1 Bladder Meridian) and say *my migraine*. Tap the side of eyebrow (#2 Gall Bladder Meridian) and say *my migraine*. Tap under the eye (#3 Stomach Meridian) and say *my migraine*. Tap under the nose (#4 Governing Vessel) and say *my migraine*.

7. Continue this sequence to points under the chin (#5 Conception Vessel), under the collarbone (#6 Kidney Meridian), under the under arm (#7 Spleen Meridian) and under the breast (#8 Liver Meridian). One round should take no longer than a minute.

8. Now repeat the sequence with the resolution: *I'm okay, and I choose to release it now.*

9. Pause now and take stock. Again, rate the intensity level of your problem from a scale of 1 to 10, 10 being the worst. Has the

pain gone up or down? If it has decreased, do a few more rounds and try to bring it even lower. By repetition, you can bring the intensity of the pain down to a manageable level, or better yet, to zero. Be aware that EFT can be practiced a few different ways, so consult the resources section for additional information.

10. Once you have mastered this sequence, you can use it anytime you're feeling stress and discomfort. It's an easy, simple technique to access your meridians and power centers, often bringing instantaneous relief.

The spiritual practices of Qigong, yoga, or EFT can be very effective tools, in your spiritual arsenal. It's important to take the time to find the spiritual tools that work for *you*.

MARIANNE JAS'S STORY: A SPIRITUAL HEALING

Esther had been treating me for months and it seemed to be working. I was feeling better and was generally optimistic about my progress. One afternoon, after finishing her pulse examination, she gently touched my arm. "Let me ask you, Marianne," she murmured, "do you believe in God?"

Okay, the g-word was unexpected. Where was she was going with this?

But Esther didn't seem to notice my self-consciousness. "What I mean to say is, do you take part in any type of spiritual practice?" she asked.

Then she leaned close. "Look, I'm not interested in what religion you are, or what spiritual belief system you hold, but my patients always do much better if they practice some sort of spiritual meditation or prayer."

As it turned out, Chinese medicine has a very specific rationale for why this is so. According to ancient texts, there is Earth and there is Heaven and humans take up the space in between. Within this relationship is a constant exchange of energy. A healthy body needs to access this energy to bring body, mind, and spirit together and complete the healing process.

Esther stood and gathered up my files. "The question I'm really asking is how much you want to take part in healing yourself. I can help a great deal in unblocking some of this emotional energy, but you are going to have to do some work on your own." She told me it didn't matter so much what I chose, a Sunday at church or a walk in nature, but I needed to open up my spiritual channels and surrender to a greater energy.

Once I thought about what she was saying I realized Esther was right. I had reached a plateau on my healing journey. My immune system was still weak and I continued to be susceptible to the same colds and infections I had suffered throughout my life.

A few days later, I found myself tentatively poking my head into the neighborhood New Age bookstore. First up, an encyclopedia of Tantric exercises. Not for me. But nearby was something intriguing, a beginner's yoga DVD. Somehow the connection that yoga provides between the body and spirit felt right for me, and I decided to give it a try. Now, eight years after that first tentative step, this practice is still a significant part of my morning ritual.

Practicing yoga gave me exactly that strong sense of inner strength, or Shen, as the Chinese call it, that Esther had been talking about. As time went on I added EFT to the agenda, complementing the other tools at my disposal. As she predicted, my energy increased, while the fatigue and minor infections nearly disappeared. Almost miraculously, I stopped getting sick.

As my Shen got stronger, I also became interested in other spiritual philosophies, incorporating the most meaningful ones into my day. As a side benefit, this also allowed me to better handle difficult situations. The emotional sale of our house, the ups and downs of being self-employed, the various and sundry family dramas—all would have been emotionally wrenching events if not for the things that yoga and other spiritual practices taught me. By sticking to a consistent meditation routine, I have been able to remain mentally and physically balanced even through the most stressful circumstances.

The most rewarding routine can eventually become rote, so every now and then I add something new to boost my Shen: paint a watercolor in the garden or sing along with an old song on the radio—anything that makes the spirit soar. By relying on these tools my Qi can flow in a smooth, uninterrupted pace, exactly what I need to stay relaxed and calm.

Inner Peace and Outer Peace

As the *Nei Jing* wisely warns us, Chinese medicine is an effective healing tool, but by itself it cannot guarantee optimum health. Acupuncture, herbs, and other therapies have proven themselves immensely successful, but to heal completely, you must learn to quiet your mind, and balance your emotions.

Take time for yourself each day. Read, meditate, or walk in the park. Tap your acupoints and bring a little color into your life. Even if it's only for a few minutes at lunch or before bed, relax and let go.

When your Qi flows, your body, mind, and emotions are at peace. Life's ups and downs become easier to deal with, and everything seems brighter. Your inner peace becomes your outer peace, and there's no better way to achieve total health.

DR. TING'S TOTAL HEALTH ESSENTIALS

5 ELEMENT CREATION CYCLE
- Fire is the mother of Earth.
- Earth is the mother of Metal.
- Metal is the mother of Water.
- Water is the mother of Wood.
- Wood is the mother of Fire.

5 ELEMENT CONTROL CYCLE
- Fire controls Metal.
- Earth controls Water.
- Metal controls Wood.
- Water controls Fire.
- Wood controls Earth.

ORGANS, ELEMENTS, AND SEASONS

- Heart–Fire–Summer
- Spleen–Earth–Late Summer
- Lungs–Metal–Autumn
- Kidneys–Water–Winter
- Liver–Wood–Spring

COLOR THERAPY

- Visualizing red benefits the Heart energy network.
- Visualizing yellow benefits the Stomach and Spleen energy network.
- Visualizing white benefits the Lung energy network.
- Visualizing blue-black benefits the Kidney energy network.
- Visualizing green benefits the Liver energy network.

OTHER SPIRITUAL TOOLS

- Qigong
- Yoga
- Feng Shui
- Emotional Freedom Technique

6

Adopt a Positive Lifestyle
How Your Habits Shape Your Health

Does this sound familiar? You drink more than you really should. You're wedded to work, staying late to answer e-mails after everyone else has gone home. Maybe you're a fast-food junkie, dependent on that Reese's rush or McNugget moment to get you through the day.

Taken individually, these activities can seem harmless, but when multiplied over a period of time, they become lifestyle choices that often have major influences on your health.

By now, the variety of things that can cause blockages in your Qi should be evident. You've read about *internal* factors, such as emotional turmoil, and you've seen the effects of *external* factors, such as weather and viruses.

But never underestimate the part that lifestyle plays in disturbing the vital flow of energy. Just as the right habits will lead to a healthy balance, the wrong ones can cause pain, malaise, discomfort and eventually disease.

Every poor lifestyle choice has the potential to drain vital energy, upsetting the Yin and Yang balance you need to maintain. The longer you continue these habits, the more your power centers absorb that imbalance and pass it along. It's a gradual spiral downward, leading to common problems such as weight gain, insomnia, and a weakened immune system.

Fortunately, you are born with a powerful ally.

Your Energy Bank Account

For thousands of years, the Chinese have equated having a strong and vital life force with owning a generous bank account. In the case of your body, that account is made up of two major currencies: **Blood** and **Qi**, both vital to lasting health.

Blood

To understand how Blood works, it's important to remember that it has both a physical and spiritual purpose, as well as a host of important characteristics:

- Blood is created by the Spleen from the foods that you eat.
- Blood gets its red color from Lungs, and the air that you breathe.
- Blood nourishes and moistens the tissues and organs.
- Blood is circulated throughout body by the Heart, and is stored in the Liver.

Rich, protein-laden Blood is full of nutrients fundamental to all facets of physical and mental health. But Blood has an even more critical function, and that is to nourish the mind, or Shen. Weak or Deficient Blood usually shows up as chronic nervousness, restlessness, or dizziness.

When someone is showing these deficient symptoms we need to strengthen the amount and flow of Blood through acupuncture and herbal treatments, followed by proper diet, rest, and meditation.

Energy Bank Account = Blood + Qi

Qi

Blood is a very visible currency, but the other half of your energy bank account, Qi, can seem much more mysterious. Qi is similar to the electricity flowing through your house. Although you can't see it, it's always there. The lights turn on, the microwave cooks, the garage door opens.

The same is true for the Qi in your body. Your Heart pumps, your Lungs take in oxygen, your Stomach digests, and your brain makes decisions. And Qi makes this all possible.

These currencies also share a mutually dependent relationship. Blood needs Qi's spark to move and circulate; Qi needs a physical place to exist, which Blood provides in the form of blood vessels. That's why Chinese medicine calls Qi the *commander* of Blood, and Blood the *mother* of Qi.

Unlike a real bank, everyone is born into the world with a certain amount of Blood and Qi already deposited, which is called *Inherited Qi*, or *Jing*. Some people start with a large bank account of Jing, others with less. The good news is that regardless of the amount of Jing a person possesses, anyone can build his or her energy assets. It's called *Acquired Qi*, and we earn it from the food we eat and the air we breathe.

Too Much Blood and Qi, or Too Little?

I can usually tell a lot about my patients' energy accounts just by watching how they sit in my waiting room. Some slump down in the chair, reading a magazine. They appear tired and depressed, nervous, or dizzy, their skin white or ashen. To me, it's obvious they are Deficient.

Deficiency is when *too little* Blood and Qi are flowing through the meridians, something I'll confirm with an examination and pulse diagnosis.

Then there are my Excessive patients. They stride in the door and immediately become impatient if they have to wait. They always seem to be overflowing with energy and can barely sit still for my office exam! They complain of being too hot no matter the temperature, and usually have a red flush on their cheeks. They have to know what's wrong and how fast I can fix them. If a medication or herbal remedy is necessary, they want it *right now*.

By and large, my Excessive patients are intelligent; have a sturdy, robust body type; and are used to wielding power and responsibility. One would think all this energy would be a good thing, but it actually has the opposite effect.

People with Excessive symptoms usually want to show the world they are balanced, so they push their bodies even harder, sometimes beyond their limits. This leads to having *too little* Qi and Blood circulating, and what is there circulating at an uneven pace. This is exactly how Qi becomes stuck and stagnates.

By the time these patients come to see me, they are facing illnesses ranging from chronic fatigue to asthma, even heart attacks. And because they can't understand why their usually strong bodies are rebelling, their frustration causes even more stress.

But illness can also be a great wakeup call. It forces people to stop and take a good look at the behavior that's causing their problem. By understanding their personal energy reserves, they can then tailor their lifestyle to match the bank account they were born with.

Now that you know your personal account exists, you can preserve and grow its assets.

Protecting Your Energy Assets

Before you can make any new deposits, you must first protect the assets that are already there. Whether big or small, your reserves of

Blood and Qi must be handled wisely. Spend recklessly, and you'll find yourself headed for bankruptcy.

Exercise	Eating Habits
Work and Rest	Social Habits

This is why reaching a balance in your lifestyle is so important. Keep your Blood and Qi plentiful and flowing and your body-kingdom's coffers will be rich with energy to spare. Live in a chronically Deficient or Excessive state, and a crash or health crisis is inevitable. To avoid this you need to make positive lifestyle choices that not only maintain a healthy equilibrium but match the energy available in your body's bank account.

This is done by balancing four all important lifestyle categories in equal amounts:

- Exercise
- Eating habits
- Social habits
- Work and rest

Each category is an essential part of life. Overdo one, or any combination, and your vital energy currency is squandered, opening the door to illness. Balancing these lifestyle activities, not only maintains the energy you already possess, but actually *adds* to your body's reserves of Blood and Qi.

Your Energy Bank Account: Maintaining Healthy Levels of Exercise

You've heard it before: Good health means a commitment to physical exercise.

When I first came to this country, I was amazed at the sheer number of gyms and exercise studios in my neighborhood. It was wonderful to see people so committed to their bodies and their health. But as a doctor I soon discovered there was another side to the fitness craze.

Underneath the desire by some to be healthy was a push to create bulky muscles and a hard body in a radically short time: *No pain, no gain.* But is that really the best thing for your body?

Certainly, physical exercise is fundamentally important to *move* Qi and Blood. When Qi remains stagnant, energy takes a dive. It would seem natural then that the more exercise you do, the more Qi you move, therefore the more energy you're building . . . right?

Not necessarily. Strong muscles are an important component of keeping you upright and flexible, yet achieving bulked-up mass by overstressing every muscle can actually make your energy system *weaker.* To achieve true physical conditioning, strengthening needs to begin from within.

Chinese medicine teaches that the emphasis should always be on the *type* and *amount* of exercise performed in relation to the Qi that is available.

Think about the strength of a lion or a cat. A lion doesn't spend hours in the gym lifting weights or pounding the treadmill. In fact, much of its time is spent lying in the shade, conserving its energy. Yet it has a natural suppleness and flexibility to leap and the reserves of strength to chase down its prey.

I tell my patients that if they want to run a marathon, they'll require a strong foundation and an inner reserve to support their training. They'll also want the ability to breathe long and deep as well as maintain strong bones and flexible joints. All of this requires a consistent flow of Blood and Qi.

There aren't any special tricks to this. Start gradually, with a daily routine that doesn't overtax your Qi reserves. The aim is to train your energy to flow in a balanced, rhythmic rate as it moves through your body.

The goal is to select a consistent exercise routine, one that can be eased into without stressing any of the major power centers.

Exercise Consistently and Make It Fun

Many people start with the best intentions. They join a gym and go all out for a few weeks. After some weightlifting, spin classes, lap swims—inevitably they become fatigued and skip a few days. Soon, a holiday rolls along and adds a few pounds to the waistline. Gradually, those intentions drift away and the gym clothes end up in the charity bin.

Whether you give up due to injury or apathy, in the end, it's easy to do more harm than good. That's why finding an activity that sparks your interests is so important—something you can do regularly, and that doesn't deplete your energy account.

How do you find that perfect activity?

One of the main reasons people don't stick to a regular routine is because it stops being fun. They start off by committing to a half hour a day on the Stairmaster, then do the same routine, day after day, until it becomes drudgery. A few months later they wonder why they couldn't make it work!

This is why adding variety is so critical. Start with a half-hour walk a couple days a week. Add a fast climb up a hill near your route. On the weekend toss a ball around with your child at the park. It's variety, not routine, that stimulates the brain. Your body will follow right along.

My grandfather, Ding Zhongying, a well-known doctor in China in his own right, was always an inspiring example to my family. Each day before seeing patients, he would do Tai Chi exercises in his room above the clinic. He would always vary the sequence, some days shorter, others longer. This was a man who never got sick, who

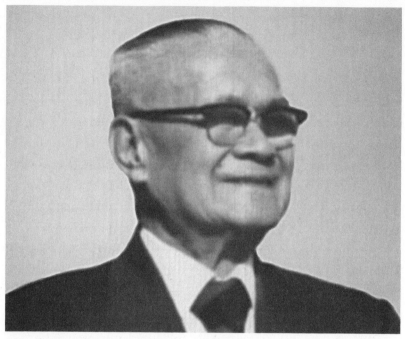

My Grandfather, Dr. Ding Zhongying

stayed strong and vital, even after moving his practice to San Francisco in his seventies. Eventually he lived to the age of ninety-three, a testament to exercising the Chinese way.

If you are hesitant about exercising alone, try it with others. Join a yoga class or find a park that offers Tai Chi or karate lessons. YMCAs and parks have swimming programs for all ages. Recently I have even changed my own routine. After twenty years of exercising alone I decided to join a gym and have taken up dancing. It gets my heart pumping, I work up a healthy sweat, and I've met many new friends.

If you have children, find some time to play with them. Pets, too. Keep in mind, though, it's always best to warm up slowly. Get the Blood and Qi circulating before any intensive movement.

Exercise According to Your Energy Type: Coming Back from Illness and Strengthening Deficiency

My patients come in all ages and shapes, and so do their energy levels. This means I need to prescribe exercise in the same way I would herbs or diet. For exercise to be effective it has to be appropriate to each individual, to *you*.

The advice I give to Deficient patients isn't particularly complicated: Get out and move. Breathe deeply. Don't sit at home and let your body fall apart. A sedentary lifestyle leads to soft muscles and tendons. Worse, it fosters Qi blockages, a sure road to illness.

Once you begin moving on a regular basis, you'll actually feel your energy channels flowing. Start with an easy twenty-minute walk down the street. Then, as your energy improves, add some additional activities, such as yoga or Pilates.

My meridian massage is another way to get your system moving. You can always work up to the activities and sports that interest you, be it jogging, biking, softball, or swimming. The main thing is to set aside at least twenty minutes a day for some kind of physical activity.

Another benefit to exercise is less obvious. When you exert yourself, your Heart pumps harder and your Lungs breathe deeper, causing your power centers to do their job more efficiently. Your Blood becomes more saturated; your digestion improves, resulting in a more acute mental state.

A note of caution: Too much exercise can be dangerous if you are new to a program, or coming back to one after illness or injury. A good rule of thumb is: Don't do too much, too soon. The important thing is to match your output of energy to your input. Eat appropriately, and incorporate periods of rest (see table 6-1).

TABLE 6-1. WEEKLY EXERCISE SCHEDULE TO STRENGTHEN DEFICIENCY

	MON	TUE	WED	THU	FRI	SAT	SUN
Internal organ exercises	15 min	15 min	15 min	15 min	15 min	Rest	Rest
Aerobic training Walk Swim	20 min (1st month) 30 min (2nd month)	Rest	20 min (1st month) 30 min (2nd month)	Rest	20 min (1st month) 30 min (2nd month)	Rest (Leisurely walk optional)	Rest (Leisurely walk optional)
Gentle cross-training Yoga (beginning) Tai Chi (beginning) Qigong (beginning) Pilates (beginning)	Rest	30 min (1st month) 1 hour (2nd month)	Rest	Rest	Rest	30 min (1st month) 1 hour (2nd month)	Rest

Exercise According to Your Energy Type: Taming Excess and Maintaining Normal Exercise Levels

Remember the Excessive person, the type who can't keep still and pushes harder no matter what? Many athletes and type A's fit this description. They train and exercise for long hours, often suffering irritability, fatigue, and injuries. If these symptoms fit you, it might be time to adjust the frequency or length of your exercise routine. Create periods of rest (Yin) between your active periods of intense exercise (Yang). Add some variety to your training routines. Instead of running ten miles, go for an easy swim. Many pro athletes are now incorporating yoga and Pilates into their training to take the edge off heavy aerobic and muscle-building regimens.

ATHLETES AND FATIGUE

Most athletes know their body well and know that rest is a critical part of performance.

A recent study by Professor David Neiman revealed that marathoners' immunity dropped sharply for three to seventy-two hours after their events. Another study by the Cooper Clinic in Dallas found that heavy physical training was linked to the suppression of white blood cells, and affected the overall health of the immune system. This is why professional athletes nearly always schedule a day of rest into the week.

When Excessive types overexercise, they risk more than just muscular injury. Too much exercise drains Blood and Qi, leaving the immune system open to viral attacks and other disease. An empty bank account is not the time to write a big check.

The spinal area is particularly susceptible to injury from overexercise. If you have a tendency to suffer from disk problems, it is generally due to a Deficiency of Blood and Qi. From a Chinese medical

TABLE 6-2. WEEKLY EXERCISE SCHEDULE FOR HEALTH MAINENANCE

	MON	TUE	WED	THU	FRI	SAT	SUN
Internal Organ Exercises	15 min	15 min	15 min	15 min	15 min	15 min	15 min
Aerobic Training Run/Jog Bike Swim Tennis or Other	30 min to 1 hour	Rest	30 min to 1 hour	Rest	30 min to 1 hour	Rest	Rest Leisurely Walk, Hike
Cross-Training Weights Yoga Pilates Tai Chi Qigong Tennis Hike Laps Swim Dance Latin Modern Ballet Ball Room		30 min		30 min			

perspective, that means the nutritious Blood and Fluids that support and bathe your muscles, tendons, and vertebrae have decreased. Here's an easy way to help your spinal fluids circulate, as well as send energy to muscles and joints. Stand with your feet about a foot apart. Bend the knees and bounce, without lifting your feet. While you are bouncing, shake your hands and then swing them gently back and forth.

To keep your energy account rich and full, it's important to balance a consistent regular exercise routine to match your body's energy level with the right amount of rest. Achieve that goal and you've found the key to a wise and sustainable health plan (see table 6-2).

HEAT INSTEAD OF ICE

For soft tissue injuries, common wisdom says that ice should be used to control the swelling. A Chinese doctor will use ice only in certain circumstances, to treat acute trauma or to stop bleeding, and then only for a short time. For stubborn injuries a Chinese practitioner will apply heat, followed by acupuncture and herbs. Long-term use of ice and application of Cold are thought to cause Stagnation of the Blood, creating more energy blockages that inhibit healing.

Your Energy Bank Account: Creating Healthy Eating Habits

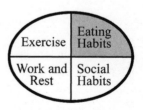

In chapter 4 you read about the healing qualities of a healthy diet. But sometimes, even if you know what to eat, you don't always choose the right things.

Often, deciding what to eat is based on flavor or cravings. People make choices according to their emotions, their mood, even what their family and friends recommend. Under these conditions it's easy to eat foods that that work against your overall health.

To eat right, you have to look at your body the way Chinese medicine does.

Your Digestive Processing Plant

The digestive organs are a great place to start. I liken them to a processing plant, working ceaselessly to mix, sort, and transform raw food and nutrients into vital Blood and Qi .

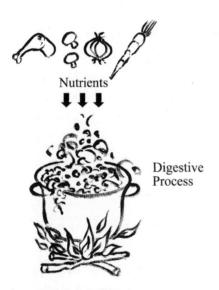

Nutrients

Digestive Process

Figure 6-1. Your Internal Digestive Processing Plant

Imagine that in the middle of your plant sits a giant pot suspended over a fire, a kind of rudimentary stove. The pot represents your Stomach, Spleen, and Small Intestine, while the fire below is fueled by the Kidneys, your body-kingdom's ministry of power (see figure 6-1).

The first stage of this digestive cooking process involves combining the basic ingredients within the pot: that is the food that you eat. As the Stomach mixes this food, it also filters and separates the nutrients. The result is then sent to the Small Intestine for further processing, before moving along to the Spleen.

Finally, the Spleen takes this soup and combines it with a key ingredient, fresh oxygen from the Lungs. It then blends the mixture into vital Blood and Qi, becoming your own nutritious essence, which your Heart then circulates via blood vessels and veins throughout your body.

Like any successful manufacturing plant, this magnificent digestive factory chugs along 24/7, combining, sorting, and producing the vital materials you need to function. But what if you neglect to provide your factory with the raw ingredients it needs to function? What happens if you let your emotions and lifestyle dictate what you eat?

Eating and Emotion

Most people have suffered an unexpected job loss or death in the family. During times like these it's not unusual for the sadness, disappointment, and fear to result in excessive drinking or eating. Considering how closely emotions are related to health, it's plain to see how these traumatic milestones can make a person too fat or too thin. Constant worry or repressed anger is often a direct cause of serious conditions such as obesity and anorexia as well as other conditions that can add up over a lifetime.

Of course people tend to focus on the most visible effects, fretting and worrying over every little pound lost or gained. But really, fluctuating weight is really just a symptom of something bigger, an indication that one's internal processing plant is not operating properly. Often it has little to do with the *amounts* a person consumes, and more to do with an unhealthy internal brew of undigested food, unprocessed emotions, retained fluids, and stagnant metabolism.

Let's say you had a stressful day. Your child has a whopping ear infection; your elderly neighbor banged his car into your fence post. On the way home from work, you stop off at the supermarket to grab a frozen dinner. But then the guy ahead in the checkout line starts fishing around for coupons and his credit card. Suddenly the frustration of the day boils into outright anger. Even though you've been snacking all day, you're famished, and you want to eat. *NOW.*

So instead of waiting until you get home, you grab that jumbo bag of M&M's and inhale handfuls as you stalk out the door.

Ahh. Feels much better, right? Wrong.

Remember the processing plant inside your digestive system? The feeling you got in the checkout line is that pot in your Stomach boiling over. The frustration and stress heat up the fire underneath, causing the pot to blow off the stove and burn everything inside.

That's what gives you the empty feeling and causes the urge to fill yourself with food—any food.

EATING AND DEPRESSION

Depression is associated with a Stagnant Liver, so avoid too many spicy foods or sweets, which create excess Heat. Instead, place a tablespoon of apple cider vinegar and a little honey in a cup of warm water and drink it three times a day. It's a great way to clear your Liver naturally, and an excellent mood changer.

Overeating and Undereating

Somehow a desire to fill up is built into food cravings—a belief that eating more will help soothe all of these daily frustrations. In reality such behavior only creates more work for the digestive system. Chinese medicine calls this condition *Stomach Fire.*

So all a person has to do is resist the cravings, right? Most of the time, it's not that simple. Any daily annoyance can be a trigger for built-up anger and frustration that goes much deeper. I see this in my patients all the time. Give emotional trauma any excuse and it will boil up from the source.

Anger, in particular, is associated with the Liver, which, is related to the Wood element. This is the same Wood that provides the fuel for the digestive pot (see figure 6-2). Unchecked, emotions of anger turn up the temperature on the stove, creating inner Heat that shows up as ravenous hunger.

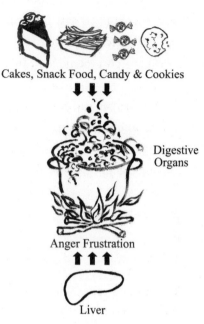

This inner Heat can also affect appetite in completely the opposite way. Although some would say there's no such thing as being "too skinny," in fact this condition is just as dangerous as being overweight.

Figure 6-2. Stomach Fire and Emotional Eating

Another effect is set into motion. When your Stomach pot boils over, gas is produced in the Blood, and the intestinal organs can fill with this gas. Now, instead of having a hollow sensation, your Stomach feels bloated and full. The smallest bite of food is unappetizing, and before long your body isn't getting the nutrients it needs to stay strong. This can lead to a loss of energy and a depressed or extremely Deficient state, and can be the root of conditions such as bulimia and anorexia.

Sluggish Organs, Sluggish Digestion

When your digestive organs slow down and are unable to transform food into nutrients or properly dispose of waste, a weakened condition results, which causes stagnation and physical blockages. Over time, a thick glue of waste is formed, which the Chinese call *Tan*. Think of Tan as a form of digestive "garbage" that becomes the building block for body fat.

That's why I jokingly refer to myself as a garbage contractor. My job is to stimulate the relevant points, to cool and clear the blockages, and kick out the Tan.

Luckily Tan *can* be removed, using acupuncture and herbal treatments. The right combination of herbs will calm the Liver, soothing pent-up anger and frustration, the actual cause of most overeating. They also help reduce bloating and gas associated with a myriad of eating disorders, release toxins through the urine and stool, and improve colon function. As a side benefit, many patients find that their moods improve and their energy increases.

Liposuction and Diet Pills: A Chinese Perspective

Many of my patients come to me depressed about their weight. Usually, by this point the Tan is so extensive that it is visible. By the time they arrive in my office they've already tried multiple diets and regimens—even liposuction—and their stories often have similar themes. At first, they have positive results—the weight drops off— but later, those extra pounds somehow seem to creep back.

This is yet another example where Chinese medicine differs in its approach.

Weight gain is not a generalized condition that can be treated using the same procedure for everyone. A weight issue is simply an indicator that your entire food processing plant needs a tune-up. Whether the cause is diet-related or stems from some combination of physical and emotional stress, the effects are the same. Your power centers have become unbalanced, and are unable to efficiently do their jobs.

We evaluate an eating disorder as a unique imbalance in each person's power centers and meridians. In other words, your weight issues are not the same as your boss's, your best friend's, or even your mother's.

By using powerful chemicals to suppress appetite and alter the flow of Qi, you are tampering with the natural energy flow through your organs and meridians. These pills or procedures may temporarily modify your body's chemistry so that you can lose weight, but they do nothing to treat the root cause of the imbalance.

This is why many of the extreme diets and weight-loss regimens often don't work. You may lose a few pounds but not realize that these formulas can also be detrimental to the intricate rhythms of your digestive organs.

Whether you "suck" the Tan out (liposuction), or use chemical diet formulas, eventually you will still have to address the root cause: the malfunction in your power centers. So before considering liposuction to lose weight, I recommend having any energy blockages looked at by a Chinese practitioner.

That's why I treat my patients with an acupuncture sequence and gentle herbal formulas that are exclusive to their specific signs and symptoms.

To succeed, weight loss requires therapy that addresses both the emotional *and* physical root of the digestion issue. Remember, calm, relaxed Blood and Qi flowing at an even pace is the ideal state. Sluggish Qi leads to sluggish decision making and poor diet choices, which can have lasting effects on your health.

So don't just look at extra weight as an unwelcome hitchhiker. Consider it a message, a way for your body to let you know you are carrying other imbalances that need to be reset.

Losing Weight by Strengthening the Power Centers: Corina

At the age of 52, Corina was overweight and unable to stand or sit for long periods of time. When I met her she was walking with a cane, heavily reliant on a number of pain medications. Eating was nearly impossible without regurgitating acid and gagging. She had been prescribed medications for a slipped disk injury and intestinal condition called gastroenterological reflux disease (GERD), but the pills had only added to the pain she was feeling. A respected paralegal and executive legal secretary, she had first been demoted, then finally forced to leave her job due to her illness.

After I examined her it was obvious that Corina was suffering from a Hot and Stagnant Liver. As we talked, the cause became clear—long-term frustration and anger stemming from her work situation. This, in turn, affected her Stomach and Spleen, which made it impossible to properly digest and transport nutrients and wastes. The resulting digestive Fire was causing a severe case of acid reflux and heartburn.

Corina had tried every diet she could get her hands on but nothing seemed to work. That didn't surprise me. She was a perfect example of someone with tired and sluggish power centers. She wasn't in the right frame of mind to make proper food and lifestyle choices. This only caused the Tan to build up and her weight to increase.

I told her it was my job to wake up her organs so that they would function normally, but for that to happen she would have to do her own part. Corina needed to figure out what was causing her anger and then forgive and forget her work-related issues.

By the time she had finished her treatment six months later, Corina had completely sworn off pain pills, and her back and esophageal reflux symptoms had disappeared. She also began a walking regimen, and reduced her dependence on sugar. The result was a loss of over thirty pounds. She even took up dancing, a hobby she had not been able to pursue for decades!

In Corina's case it wasn't her weight that caused the problem. The weight was a *side effect* of the imbalance in her power centers, the real culprit behind her illness. Once her body was functioning normally, the pounds dropped away and her digestion went back to its normal function.

How to Create Healthy Eating Habits

In chapter 4 we discussed the power of food to heal illness and disease. But how can you create a lifelong eating regimen that sustains you on a daily basis?

It comes back to making healthy eating habits, and being aware of the effects these habits create. The road to great health is built on maintaining an evenly balanced energy flow. By creating random spikes and surges, this flow is interrupted, affecting your energy system in negative ways.

For example, a spicy chicken enchilada may seem irresistible. But if your body is running Hot from stress and frustration, the Heat generated from the spices only conspires to bring your Blood and fluids to a boil. Continue with this sort of diet and the accumulated Heat will eventually dry you out.

Maybe you can't help dipping into that tub of Haagen-Dazs in the freezer. Remember that frozen foods such as ice cream take an enormous amount of energy to heat up and digest. In addition, sugar causes the digestive system to work overtime, so if you're already experiencing exhaustion, too much ice cream can cause your Qi to drain away.

It's not just rich and exotic treats that should be avoided; some of the worst culprits are the simple things people eat habitually every day.

Creating Healthy Eating Habits: Sugar

When I took my first look at supermarkets in this country, I was amazed not only at the variety of foods available, but at how many of these products contain sugar in one or another form. Unfortunately, many digestive problems and diseases are directly caused by over-consuming those sugar-heavy foods.

If you habitually eat *large* servings of foods with a high sugar content, you are putting too much of a powerful substance into your power centers.

Refined (white) sugar and such processed ingredients such as high-fructose corn syrup, in particular, create extra work for the Spleen, sending Stomach fluids and enzymes into overdrive. This leads to an excess of Heat and often causes bloating, gas, and a drop in energy. Although it seems like you're getting a burst of energy, in fact it's only a temporary spike. That feeling can't be maintained because it's not coming from true nutritional storehouses of energy.

Other common results of eating too much sugar are bad breath, migraine headaches, and mouth sores. All of these are clues that you may be suffering from Stomach Fire, or a Heat condition that is best treated with a combination of herbs, acupuncture, and cooling foods.

Fortunately, there are alternatives to refined sugar. In fact, I believe a small amount of raw organic or brown sugar can actually be a beneficial part of your daily diet. In China, raw sugar is used medicinally to soothe sore throats and ease the symptoms of chronic diarrhea. Mixed with water, it also has been known to revive someone after fainting.

An even better choice is to drip some honey or molasses on your bowl of oatmeal, a healthy way to settle those sugar cravings. Remember a little bit of refined sugar is a nice treat but a little goes a long way.

Creating Healthy Eating Habits: Salt

Salt is a cooling mineral and, if used moderately, is helpful to your ministry of power, the Kidneys. If overused in a processed form, however, salt can be a devastating substance, causing water retention, high blood pressure, and weakened bones. Take a good look at the box of crackers you are about to buy. You'll be surprised at how much salt is listed there. Packaged and processed foods are simply loaded with it. Since recommended salt consumption can vary greatly from individual to individual, I always advise eating salt in modest amounts and in its purest form. Sea salt, for instance, is an excellent natural way to get the same taste without the chemicals.

Creating Healthy Eating Habits: Caffeine

Who doesn't go through the day and crave a quick pick-me-up? It's not easy to resist the allure of a steaming hot mocha, or the cooling sweetness of an ice-cold soda. Try to resist. Just like sugar, excess caffeine creates an explosion of Heat and Excessive Yang energy that sends your power centers spiraling out of control. That extra-tall morning mocha can act as a double whammy, mixing two of the Five Temperature Devils: Heat (sugar and caffeine) and Damp (milk and whipped cream). Some of these ingredients are also present in popular high-energy drinks.

Why do so many people crave caffeine? Because their energy bank is sending them signals that their Qi account is low, and only that burst of caffeine will fill the coffers. In actuality they are creating artificial jolts that only force their power centers to artificially speed up their work.

The Kidneys, in particular, jump into hyper drive, and before long they are working overtime. This expresses itself in headaches, fatigue, and eventual adrenal exhaustion.

Some people have strong energy reserves and a moderate amount of caffeine isn't a problem. If, however, you *routinely* feel tense or suffer from fatigue, it could be that caffeine is draining your energy.

What's the right amount? Like everything else you put in your body, beverages that contain caffeine should be drunk in moderation, if at all. Coffee has the most milligrams per ounce of caffeine, whereas black teas, hot chocolate, and sodas contain about half that amount. By sticking to one small cup of plain coffee per day, most people will be fine. But if you find yourself drinking multiple servings of caffeinated, sugary drinks throughout the day, it might be time to reconsider.

This is especially true if you are experiencing symptoms relating to the Kidneys, thyroid problems, backaches, weak knees or legs, dark circles underneath your eyes, or an aversion to cold. Symptoms of a disrupted Liver network include headaches; red eyes, face, or skin; and insomnia.

To kick the caffeine habit, create an energy boost in a more natural way, using exercise or a healthy meal. Another option is coffee substitutes, such as Cafix or Dacopa, as well as decaffeinated coffee or tea. Green tea is a good choice, too. It's hot in temperature but actually has a cooling effect on the body and is a wonderful antioxidant.

CAFFEINE AND MISCARRIAGE

If you are trying to conceive or if you're already pregnant, and you constantly feel exhausted, it's a good idea remove caffeine from your diet. Exhaustion usually means you do not have enough Blood or Qi to sustain the fetus.

I also recommend an energy diagnosis from a reputable Chinese practitioner in your area. My practice has had much success in nourishing and strengthening the body before and during pregnancy.

Creating Healthy Eating Habits: Chocolate

Let's just say it. There aren't a lot of things on earth tastier than a morsel of chocolate. Indulging every now and then is one of life's great treats, especially if it's dark chocolate. It's high in antioxidants and a beneficial food for certain health risks. Remember, though, that chocolate *also* contains refined sugar, caffeine, and dairy products. By adding powdered chocolate to a caffeinated coffee drink, then combining it with milk, whipped cream, and sugar, you are doubling the amount of white sugar and caffeine going into your system. Again, it's your Liver and Kidneys that take the brunt of this onslaught, so make chocolates and chocolate-flavored products a sporadic treat and enjoy!

Know Your Body, Know Yourself

When my patients ask me how to change their eating habits, I tell them it starts when they become aware of their body.

The easiest way to start regulating and strengthening your power centers is by eating healthy foods that match your energy and temperature type. I generally recommend an easy-to-digest, protein-rich

TABLE 6-3. SAMPLE MENU

Your Symptoms	Healing Foods	Sample Menu
If experiencing **Hot** symptoms	Eat Cold, Cooling, and/or Neutral foods	Breakfast: Egg white, citrus fruit Lunch: Pork or beef, potato, carrots, sweet rice Dinner: Cucumber salad, lettuce, watermelon
If experiencing **Cold** symptoms	Eat Hot, Warming, and/or Neutral foods	Breakfast: Eggs, ham, mango Lunch: Lamb, squash with nutmeg Dinner: Chicken and onion soup
If experiencing **Damp** symptoms	Eat Drying and/or Neutral foods	Breakfast: Jasmine tea, eggs Lunch: Pork and cabbage Dinner: Barley soup, 3-bean salad, parsley
If experiencing **Dry** symptoms	Eat Lubricating and/or Neutral foods	Breakfast: Cottage cheese, yogurt Lunch: Clam chowder Dinner: Spinach omelet with strawberries
If experiencing **Excessive** symptoms	Eat Neutral foods	Breakfast: Eggs, peaches Lunch: White fish and sweet rice Dinner: Carrot salad, fruit
If experiencing **Deficient** symptoms	Eat Strengthening and/or Neutral foods	Breakfast: Oatmeal with bananas, dates, figs Lunch: Liver and onions Dinner: Chicken and asparagus

diet, rather than relying on too many simple and processed carbohydrates. Protein takes a lot longer to digest, and offers a bigger energy boost. Foods high in simple carbs, such as sugar and white flour products, do not provide sufficient energy to your bank account because they are so easily absorbed into the blood stream. Instead, eat a helping of complex carbohydrates made up of whole grains, legumes, and starchy and leafy green vegetables.

A good place to start is the food and temperature charts (see pages 100–101) and my Sample Menu (see table 6-3). These guidelines will help you begin to make the right choices.

Changing any habit, eating or otherwise, involves a variety of physical and emotional factors. You have already read about ways to relieve stress through meditative exercises as well as visualization and EFT (see chapter 3). As it happens, these are also very effective ways to stop those destructive cravings.

EFT in particular has proved to be very effective in many cases. The basic sequence is the same: rate the intensity of your craving from 1 to 10, then create an easy phrase that describes your predicament. An example might be: *Even though I am so stressed and I just can't stop snacking, drinking caffeine/sugar/etc., I accept myself, or I'm taking care of myself and I choose to release this craving now.* Get creative, and really voice your concerns while you tap your acupoints. If you're interested in finding out more about specialized EFT programs and techniques, check the resources section or the Internet for more support.

Your Energy Bank Account: Balancing Your Social Habits

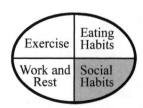

Just about everyone's social habits begin when they're young. Important signals come from all over, and sometimes life is filled with all the wrong cues. Parents or relatives may favor a daily mug of beer or a martini to relax. Best friends drag one another to the parking lot for that cigarette "you just *have* to try." And who doesn't remember those nights that lasted until the sun came up. Many also grow up with unhealthy cultural customs that can have lasting effects.

It's a heady brew of temptation and taste, one that can eventually become locked into persistent behavior. After a while, some people don't even think twice about having a couple cigarettes at lunch, or a six-pack after work.

But they should.

Chinese medicine considers social habits to be an essential part of maintaining proper health. Even as early as 200 BC the wise words of the *Nei Jing* contained passages commenting on the unhealthy impact of alcoholism and social excesses on society.

A few glasses of wine at night may not seem like a big deal, but if you are habitually tense, the temporary relaxation wine brings actually causes *more* internal Heat. This can lead to a downward spiral of chronic sluggishness, headaches, and muddled thinking. Please recognize that *whatever* you put into your body it will affect your Qi and power centers. The wrong foods always have the potential to disrupt and drain your energy bank account, particularly when consumed in excess or without regard to the effects.

Balancing Your Social Habits: Alcohol

For many people the good life means the occasional glass of beer, wine, or maybe a frosty margarita. The good news is that a little bit of alcohol can actually help boost your Blood flow and circulation.

Here again, quantity matters. Alcohol works much the same as sugar. It's classified as a Hot and Damp substance, so when a swig of beer goes down, it creates a temporary burst of energy, known as "the buzz," What you can't feel is the excess Heat in your body, especially in your Liver. This combination of Heat and Dampness makes the Qi and Blood in your meridians become sluggish, and can cause blockages and Stagnation, evident as patches of purple discoloration on the cheeks and nose of heavy drinkers.

Some people use alcohol as a way to lift their spirits. From a Chinese perspective, feelings of loneliness or depression mean that some of the power centers or meridians are blocked, and that Qi is not moving freely. When people use alcohol as a way to move this stagnant emotional energy, they don't realize it is actually having a damaging effect on their Qi.

This is why controlling the amount of alcohol you drink is so vital to your health. And if you are someone who runs Hot, it's especially important. When Heat increases inside that pot on your inner stove, it has no place to vent except into the power centers. Overindulging, especially in hard liquor, causes serious systemic problems in the Liver. These include chronic headaches and dizziness, which can easily escalate to more serious symptoms such as aggression and violent behavior.

If your Qi needs to be jump-started, there are ways other than alcohol to light up its energy channels. My internal organ exercises, for example, or some Qigong, can be an excellent tool; so is acupuncture, or even a round of EFT that focuses on your cravings (see pages 142–146). Once Qi is flowing easily and naturally, my patients usually find it easier to skip that second Mai Tai. By following nature's way, the body gets the emotional support it needs, without damaging precious organs. Remember: By using alcohol to self-medicate, your symptoms will only get worse until you find other ways to release those feelings of anger, fear, and anxiety.

If your alcohol consumption has become a problem, and you are considering counseling or a recovery program, a Chinese medical diagnosis can be an effective addition. Acupuncture and herbs have proven themselves to be effective treatment, while working in tandem with many addiction recovery programs. (Please refer to the resources section for more details.)

Balancing Your Social Habits: Tobacco

Like sugar and caffeine, tobacco smoke is also energetically Hot, and this is the kind of Heat that stagnates in the Lungs. Most smokers are aware of the dangers of nicotine, but not of Lung Stagnation. Instead, they enjoy the warm rush of Heat speeding throughout their body, not realizing that the energetic high it creates can have devastating effects. In China we say that long-term cigarette smoke "cooks" the Lung organ and its meridians. The Heat and Dry Devils are particularly damaging to one's internal organ system, adding to the problems of emphysema and cancer.

This is the reason Chinese medicine takes the position that one cigarette a month is one cigarette too many. As with alcohol, you can fight your cravings for tobacco products by using some of the healthy ways we've discussed to reduce their use and get your Qi moving and flowing.

Balancing Your Social Habits: Drugs

Chinese medicine has long analyzed the effects of drugs and drug addiction. The cultivation of opium and heroin in early eighteenth-century China resulted in widespread drug use, and this in turn led to a quest by doctors to understand the drugs' effects on the body's power centers.

What they discovered was just how pervasively these drugs can transform nearly every organ in the body.

This is especially true today, with prescription and recreational drugs being formulated in ever more potent variations. Many are so powerful they enter all fourteen meridians, altering the flow and direction of Qi.

These medications have proven indispensable when prescribed for great pain, injury, or devastating illness, and there is no doubt they have played a critical role in saving lives. However, if you have been using strong drugs for extended periods, and your emotional and physical symptoms have *not* improved, it may be time to reevaluate these prescriptions, particularly if you are regularly adding alcohol to the mix.

There's no way to dress up this topic. When used for extended periods of time, especially recreationally or without supervision, drugs can cause extreme damage to your Liver and Kidneys, draining the precious Inherited Qi in your bank account. How does this happen?

Like herbs and foods, drugs have their own temperature and properties. Opioids (narcotics) for example, tend to be very active (Yang). Initially they are warm and drying and act like a Heat Devil. Later, however, these drugs can cause the body to cool, causing shakes and shivers. These swings from Hot to Cold can add up over long periods of drug use, causing one's power centers to break down and become unable to do their job.

One of the most insidious effects of long-term drug use is the blockage it causes in the Heart meridian. This obstruction isn't just physical; the spirit, or Shen, is deeply affected, leaving a person without a healthy, vibrant king. The ability to stay aware and make decisions breaks down, upsetting the intricate balance of energy within the body-kingdom. This is why there is so much mental confusion and disturbed thinking in drug-addicted people.

As a Chinese doctor, I am always distressed to see the sheer number of overdoses caused by prescription drugs. Unfortunately, overly optimistic advertising messages are not helping matters. It is an unnecessary tragedy. Chinese medicine offers more natural ways to confront illness, methods that avoid exposing one's systems to powerful drugs.

This is accomplished by following the same treatment patterns used for many other illnesses. I look at my patients according to their specific energy pattern, then assess and treat their physical and emotional weaknesses. By identifying the root cause, the patients can then be slowly weaned from their habit.

Prescription Drugs and Depression: Mary

A few years ago, Mary, 55, came to me seeking help to reduce the multiple medicines she was taking for depression. She had been having suicidal tendencies and severe panic attacks, and had been under continual psychiatric care. But the years of prescription medications were only making her life more miserable.

When I first saw Mary, her panic attacks had returned full force, leaving her incapacitated for days. She believed the drugs were losing their strength and causing insomnia and debilitating disorientation. Her doctor had already ordered a blood test to see whether there was any Liver or Kidney damage, something I had also suspected when I examined her. Insomnia and exhaustion are often a telling sign of a severely weakened Kidney and Liver.

As with most chronic diseases, long-term drug use can't be stopped overnight. For Mary to get better we managed to gently wean her from her medications as gently as possible, which were then reduced over the ensuing months. Every few weeks we incrementally lowered the dosage of her medications one pill at a time, watching carefully for any negative effects. I also prescribed a daily round of herbs and meridian exercises, which she regularly performed.

Slowly Mary's weak and sluggish organs came back to life, and within four months they had returned to their healthy function. By the end of the year, Mary no longer needed her medications, and she had become completely symptom free. Best of all, she has experienced no mental depression or panic attacks since she left my care. Mary's body is once again functioning in the way nature intended.

Balancing Your Social Habits: Sex

Sex is part of the fabric of life, the most intimate way people show love to one another. But as described in Chinese medicine, it is also considered a lifestyle *habit*. And just like eating and exercise habits, indulging in too much or too little sex can be a sign of other imbalances.

Engaging in an intimate sexual relationship is actually stimulating a powerful healing response in the body-kingdom. This is because the meridians of all five power centers pass through and along the sexual organs.

This is especially true of the Heart, which holds emotions of joy, love, and passion. When you hold your partner in an intimate embrace, energy moves along the meridian highways directly to the Heart. These powerful emotions are then released and flood through the body, nourishing and fortifying both physically and spiritually.

But you share much more than just emotional energy when you are engaged in the sexual act. You are exchanging one of your most powerful essences—your Jing, or inherited Qi. Jing, as you know, is a crucial substance in your human existence. What is also important to know is that Jing is passed from one person to another within bodily fluids, making it one of your most revered treasures. Not only does Jing carry the foundation for an embryo's growth, it is the vessel that holds your DNA. Fixed at birth, Jing stays with you throughout your lifetime.

Jing is affected and exchanged with sexual activity, but it has other functions within the body as well. It is the key to healthy bones, teeth, even brain growth—nearly every part of the aging process. Jing Qi resides in the Kidneys, which is why keeping that organ healthy and strong is so critical for a fulfilling sex life.

Sex: Too Much or Too Little?

For good sex a person needs a functioning power plant. For great sex that power plant has to be running at peak capacity. When it's not, many people experience embarrassing or upsetting interruptions such as a loss of libido, erectile dysfunction, or painful intercourse. This is an obvious sign that the Kidneys are not producing enough Blood and Fluids, a clue that the body may be Deficient.

If you find yourself listless, with no appetite for sex, your Kidneys are telling you it's time for an energy tune-up. Add kidney beans, black beans, sardines, and walnuts to your diet. For men, an occasional serving of shrimp can heighten potency and desire. And for additional strengthening, rub the Bladder points along your lower back as well as the Kidney points underneath your collarbone at least three times a day (see figure 6-3).

THE FIRST SEX EXPERTS

The Chinese were one of the first to publish a text outlining the effects of sex on health. The *Nei Jing*, *The Classic of the Plain Girl* and *The Counsels of a Simple Girl* all advocate that people should balance sexual activity as an important part of staying healthy.

In fact, if one's body is healthy and well-maintained, traditional Chinese medicine advocates having sex well into one's nineties!

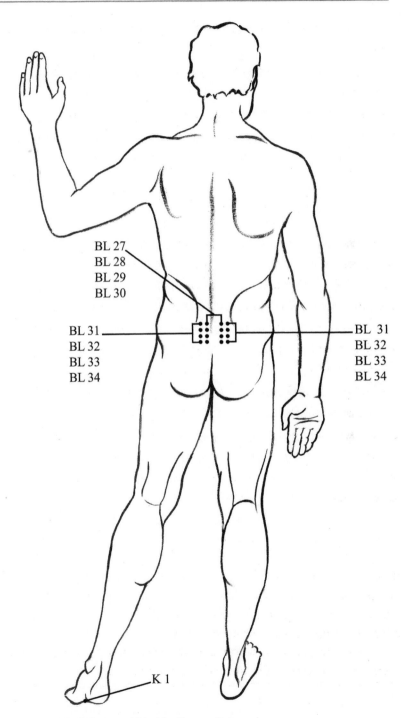

Figure 6-3. Kidney and Bladder Energy Points

Of course, not everyone suffers from lack of desire. Some have the opposite condition: They can't seem to have enough sex, no matter what. Constant cravings like these mean that there is too much Heat in the body. Somehow it all has to vent, and the act of intercourse becomes the pathway.

This Excessive Heat is related to a number of things: diet, repressed emotion, and excessive alcohol and/or drug consumption. If this fits you, try removing Hot foods from your diet, as well as caffeine and alcohol, and see if your symptoms improve.

Many people believe there is no such thing as too much sex, but an addiction to intimate encounters drains the Jing and can actually cause premature aging. How much is too much? If you're middle aged and you still need multiple sexual encounters every day, it's a clue that your body-kingdom is overheated and imbalanced.

Fortunately, Chinese medicine can treat extreme sexual problems and has had great success with everything from impotence to erectile dysfunction.

Sex is a wonderful part of human relationships and a beautiful expression of intimacy. Just as with other lifestyle habits, moderation is the key. If you take care of your body and eat well, you'll have the energy to maintain an active sex life into your eighties and beyond.

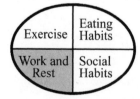

Your Energy Bank Account: The Balance Between Work and Rest

It's Saturday night and you started work at six in the morning. Now it's midnight and you're still at your job. The family went to bed hours ago yet you still feel obligated to do everything asked of you, even tasks that could be put off until Monday.

It isn't very hard to spot the signs of a workaholic. I see it in my practice all the time. Patients will come in with an ailment, then ask me to fix them up so they can continue working the same grinding schedule. "I don't have time to think about myself," they'll say.

How can they, when they are perennially drained and exhausted?

Beside poor diet, exercise, and other lifestyle habits, overwork is one of the most influential factors contributing to illness. Your work habits need to be balanced, or exhaustion and other health-related problems are bound to crop up.

In years past there have been a number of high-profile examples. You might recall one of television's most beloved news anchors dying quite suddenly of a massive coronary attack at age fifty-eight. Diagnosed with heart issues some years prior, he was known for putting in fourteen-hour days, even squeezing in a regular aerobic workout.

Whether it was running the news division, preparing for his weekly news show, or the dealing with the wear and tear of a 24-hour news cycle, this was a man known for his upbeat energy and relentless dedication.

Tragically, it all added up to a work-rest relationship that was way out of balance: a prime example of what can happen when a power center (the Heart) is signaling distress, yet a highly driven work ethic is driving the body past what it can absorb. By continuing to expend excessive energy throughout the day and into the evening, it's easy to produce a complete breakdown of the entire energy network.

To protect your power centers against excessive wear and tear, it's so important to carefully conserve and spend your bank account of Blood and Qi. The way I put it to my patients is that they must "save their money" by creating the right balance of work and rest.

Simplify Your Life

For many people the breakneck pace of modern life can be overwhelming. Kids, jobs, commutes, activities—I'm often amazed at the hectic schedules my patients keep. When they ask me how to reduce this stress and fill up their energy reserves, my answer is simple, and it doesn't cost a thing.

Slow down. Cut out nonessential activities, find a carpool to share the driving, ask your boss for permission to complete some work at home—anything to ease the pressure and give your body the chance it needs to renew those depleted reserves.

Blood and Qi are the most valuable commodities you own. Without this energy currency, you have little hope of accomplishing anything. By slowing the frenzied pace you are adding income to your energy bank account, making it easier to achieve the goals you desire.

This might sound simplistic, but you'd be amazed how few people want to make these changes. Loving your body means taking a rest every now and then. It means recognizing that you need healthy amounts of exercise and food. By treating yourself like a battered Volvo, you'll only get weaker. Continue to push yourself beyond the limits, and you open yourself up to volatile emotions that can wreak havoc with the immune system. Remember, the more your body breaks down, the more it will cost to repair, just like that old Volvo.

If this advice sounds unrealistic, ask yourself this—how rewarding is life if you don't have the energy to live it?

Physical work is a good example. Let's say you work at a garden center and part of your duties involves lifting heavy bags of soil in and out of cars all day. The exertion of heavy lifting can exhaust your Lung Qi, leaving you winded and weakening the immune system.

The same is true for mental exertion. If you stay up all night staring at a tax program, you are draining your Spleen Qi when it should be rebuilding and regenerating.

Weakening these organs affects your ability to digest food and nutrients, leading to sizable withdrawals of Blood and Qi from your energy bank account.

The Art of Balance

In these hectic times, my patients sometimes accuse me of being unrealistic. For many, the concept of rest seems a rare and decadent luxury. It's not that difficult, however, if you make a few simple changes.

If your job requires you to sit in front of a computer for long hours, stop and take a break every now and then. Get up and stretch, breathe deeply, move around. This not only keeps your muscles from stagnating but ensures that your Blood and Qi circulate. Try massaging your head, scalp, and ears; and pat the meridians in your legs and feet.

If you perform a lot of physical work, your body needs those periodic breaks even more. Find a comfortable place to rest and take the strain off your knees and back. This is a good way to balance some of that accumulated Yang energy and move into a Yin state. After lunch I always take a five- or ten-minute rest to help my power centers digest. It regenerates the Blood and Qi I need, and, as a side benefit, gives my mind some time off.

One of my Heart patients came up with an innovative solution to his frantic schedule: He brought a couch to his workplace, so he could stretch out whenever the stress became too much.

By committing to fifty-hour workweeks and late nights at the office it's not always possible to get the rest you need. Be creative. Juggle the ingredients within your work environment. Whatever it takes to keep that energy account topped off. The more you aim for a healthy balance between Yin and Yang, the better chance you have of keeping illness at bay.

Rebuilding an Energy Deficit: Marcia

Marcia arrived in my office with a severe sinus condition that had plagued her for decades. She had three children, was involved in several charities, and did all the housework. No wonder she was feeling completely overwhelmed. When I asked about her lifestyle, Marcia confided that she skipped meals, got little rest, and had no time for herself.

I gently let her know that she was draining her energy bank account, creating a deficit that eventually would be hard to replenish. The best thing she could do was to sit down with her children, eat three balanced meals a day, and go to bed at a reasonable hour, even if that meant leaving the dishes until the next morning. Finally, I suggested hiring a weekly maid service until she had gathered enough energy to tackle her own housework.

Marcia did all of these things, and after a few weeks of acupuncture sessions and a daily regimen of herbs, her sinus condition disappeared.

Stretching out and delegating responsibility made a big difference in Marcia's life. By honoring her body and simplifying a few daily tasks, she replenished her energy reserves and came back stronger than ever.

In a way, your system is a lot like a cranky computer's. When your body suddenly freezes up, the only way to get it running again is to reboot. Sometimes your body just need to shut down, unplug, and start all over again.

Too Much Rest

Most people think the dangers lie in overtaxing their body, not realizing that the opposite condition is equally damaging. Believe it or
not, too much rest can also be hazardous to your health.

For every person who clocks in at the office or climbs a telephone
pole, there are others who are retired or live independently from
other forms of income. Even without the responsibilities of a career,
many of these patients have become sedentary or lost their desire to
be active.

By spending day after day lounging around the pool or in other
listless pursuits, they have effectively disengaged their body and
their mind. Precious Qi is being wasted by too little movement, resulting in sluggishness and organ dysfunction. Energy stagnates,
muscles weaken, and injury is more likely.

For these patients, it's important to keep the Qi moving and flowing, and to stay open and active to the world around them.

I generally recommend my meridian exercises as well as some
sort of fun hobby or pastime that gets them up and moving—charity
work, taking a class, or even volunteering at the local library.

Cutting Out the Extremes

Who doesn't crave a recipe for the perfect lifestyle? People often ask
me, "How much should I eat? . . . How long should I work? . . . How
much should I exercise?"

The answers aren't always easy. Maintaining a proper balance can
be a delicate process. But the simple answer is to keep life as uncom-
plicated as possible, and follow nature's way.

Everything in life is a choice—*your* choice. In my experience anyone can choose a healthy habit over a less healthy one.

Next time you're in the gym, think about a rest before pushing twenty more repetitions on the weight machine. Check your personal energy reserves and be honest about what you really need. Don't think that small piece of toast can carry you through the morning or that doubling your medication will make you feel better faster. Be aware of when you feel overly tense or exhausted, and make the right decisions about rest and recovery.

It all comes down to Blood and Qi. If it's plentiful and flowing, there will be energy to spare. But if you feel weak, or if your energy is surging out of control, it's time to make those lifestyle changes that will guarantee your body's energy bank account remains even.

Exercise, diet, work, rest, and social habits—a rich and meaningful life includes a moderate amount of each of these activities.

You don't have to be overly rigid. Eat well, breathe deeply, avoid excessive stress, live in harmony with your environment, give yourself the time to quiet your mind, and you'll have created a healthy place for your Blood and Qi to thrive.

DR. TING'S TOTAL HEALTH ESSENTIALS

YOUR ENERGY BANK ACCOUNT = BLOOD + QI

Blood

- **Blood** is created by the Spleen from the foods that you eat.
- **Blood** gets its red color from the Lungs, and the air that you breathe.
- **Blood** nourishes and moistens your tissues and organs.
- **Blood** is circulated throughout body by your Heart, and is stored in your Liver.

Qi

- **Inherited Qi (Jing)** is inherited at birth.
- **Acquired Qi** is created through your lifestyle

THE KEY TO A HEALTHY LIFE IS A BALANCE AMONG THESE FOUR LIFESTYLE CATEGORIES

- **Exercise:** Tailor exercise to your energy type:
  - **Deficient Conditions** (do the Internal Organ exercises daily, walk three times weekly, cross-train once weekly, take three days off)
  - **Health Maintenance** (do the Internal Organ exercises daily, aerobic exercises four times weekly, cross-train twice weekly, take one day off)
- **Eating Habits:** Sluggish power centers will result in sluggish digestion and weight issues. To create healthy eating habits:
  - Find ways to balance your stress before you eat.
  - Eat the right foods for your energy type.
  - Moderate your intake of sugar, salt, caffeine, and chocolate.
- **Social Habits:** Healthy social habits are essential to good health. Enjoy alcohol, drugs, and sex in moderation.
  - **Alcohol:** Moderate amounts boost Blood flow and circulation. Too much alcohol creates excess Heat in the body, leading to chronic physical and behavioral changes.
  - **Tobacco:** "Cooks" the Lung and its meridians. To be avoided at all costs.
  - **Drugs:** The use of recreational drugs upsets the balance of Qi and can be hazardous. Prescription drugs should be used only according to a doctor's guidelines. If no results are seen over a long period, their use should be reevaluated.
  - **Sex:** A powerful healing connection, sexual intercourse should be enjoyed in moderation. Too many sexual encounters can deplete your Qi and Jing.
- **Work and Rest:** Create a daily balance between work and rest.

7

Maximize Your Energy
Tuning In to Sun and Seasons

It's a clear summer day and you're sitting on a sandy beach. Far out at sea, something catches your eye—a ripple on the surface. Racing along the ocean floor, it gathers energy, reaching its peak height, before crashing magnificently onto the shore. It's a single wave, one of countless more, part of an endless cycle that repeats itself millions of times on every beach in the world.

A wave is just one of nature's many cycles, a rise and fall of energy that is shared by every form of life on the planet. Trees lose their leaves and grow new ones; crops grow, mature, and lie fallow; animals hibernate and awaken in spring. Humans, too, are part of this continuous cycle of nature, our bodies generating personal waves of energy or Qi, which rise, crest, and crash. Work against these daily and seasonal cycles, manage them improperly, and it's easy to attract everything from mild ailments to serious illness.

Fortunately, there are a number of ways to stay in tune with nature.

The internal and external energy rhythms of every organ and meridian are finely attuned to solar and lunar cycles. By paying close attention to these patterns, anyone can maximize one's energy and, as a result, keep one's immune system poised to fight invaders.

Nature's Clock

When I began seeing patients as a young doctor in Shanghai many years ago, I suddenly found myself faced with a very hectic lifestyle.

I was newly married, and, as was customary, had moved in with my in-laws across town. In addition to a heavy patient load at the hospital, my household chores had doubled. It was a busy time, yes, but I also tried to keep a rhythm and consistency to my day.

At sunrise, we would wake up and go to the local markets to shop for food. I would make a hearty breakfast for my family, then bicycle for forty-five minutes to the hospital. When 8:00 a.m. rolled around, my colleagues and I finished our communal Guang Bo exercises and then began seeing patients.

After a long day, I would bicycle home with the setting sun, arriving in time to help with dinner and catch up with my family before bed. It was a full schedule but one that kept my body in tune with nature.

I now live halfway around the world, and my daily schedule remains very much the same. I still get up at sunrise and do my exercises. Since my office is only a short distance from where I live, I usually walk to work. At the end of the day, it's another brisk walk home and a light supper before bed.

Today I am almost seventy-two years old, but by following this daily cycle, I'm able to work six days a week and am healthier and more rested than some of my younger patients.

When asked how I do it, I always say the same thing: Pay attention to the sky above and the body within.

Your Daily Yin and Yang Cycle

I've talked about the opposing energies of Yin and Yang and how critical it is to keep them balanced. There is no better example of this than your body's 24-hour solar and lunar cycles (see figure 7-1). The sun represents a hot active, Yang energy; the moon, a cold and restful Yin energy. For optimal health, these two opposing energies must be balanced, even amid hectic daily schedules.

Chinese medicine considers our daily activities—eating, sleeping, working, and playing—to be best suited to specific times of the day. (Note that these are approximate times since sunrise and sunset vary at different times of the year.)

- **Rising Yang:** Each morning the sun rises at approximately **6:00 a.m.**, the beginning of the Yang cycle. This is the time when your organs and circulatory systems wake up and begin digesting the food and creating the oxygen that will power you through the day.
- **Peak Yang:** At **12:00 p.m.** the sun reaches what we call "Peak Yang." During this time your body is at its maximum energy level, and is ready for all activities. Following noon, the Yin cycle begins to take effect.
- **Rising Yin:** From **3:00 to 6:00 p.m.** the sun is descending and the moon begins to rise. Even though these hours are still active ones, the body is starting to get ready for rest.
- **Peak Yin:** During the early evening, from **6:00 p.m. to 12:00 a.m.**, your organs wind down, finally reaching the "Peak Yin," or full rest, at midnight. While you sleep, your power centers begin rebalancing themselves.
- **Rising Yang:** As **3:00 a.m.** rolls around, Yin is transitioning back into Yang, and by sunrise the body is once again in the

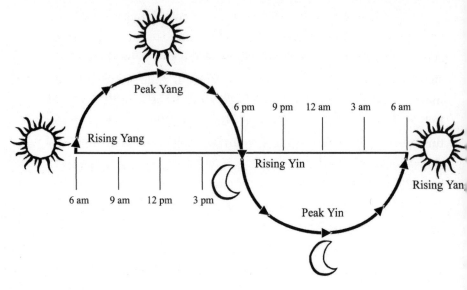

Figure 7-1. Daily Yin and Yang Cycle

Yang phase. The cycle has gone full circle and you are ready for a new day.

Your Daily Body Clock

In addition all of nature's cycles going on outside the body, human beings share a matching rhythm inside our body-kingdom. It's as regular as the sun rising and setting; an internal clock ticking away inside everyone.

It works like this: Every Zhang or Yin organ and its related Fu or Zi partner has a particular time of day that it is most active and best able to do its job. The five power centers and partner organs peak at two-hour intervals, giving each organ its own special time to shine.

By paying attention to those peaks, it's easier to understand what your power centers are saying at certain times of the day. For instance, if you are chronically tired late in the afternoon, it may be a sign that the Bladder or Kidneys are weak. If concentrating in the morning hours is difficult, it can be due to a weak digestive system. In both cases your power centers are talking back to you through nature's clock. To evaluate these symptoms, a Chinese doctor will consider the time of day they occur, then will treat the cause before it becomes a major health problem.

The following sections will show you how to synchronize your daily schedule to nature's rhythms. Once you become attuned to these external and internal energy cycles, you can begin to make smarter lifestyle choices that will optimize your overall health.

Dawn: Lungs

Your **Lungs** function at their highest capacity in the predawn hours from **3:00 to 5:00 a.m.** Remember, this organ is your Qi leader, in charge of respiration and keeping the immune system strong.

When you get up in the morning, look and listen to your body. Pay attention to the signs and your Lungs will often show you what they are experiencing.

3:00 to 5:00 a.m.—Lungs

Do you cough a lot? Are you overly thirsty? Do you take long, deep breaths or shallow, short ones? Remember that in Chinese medicine, your nose is considered the gateway to the Lungs. If you are regularly

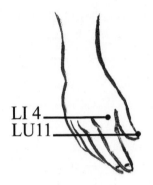

LI 4
LU11

Figure 7-2. Strengthen your Lung meridian along acupoints *Large Intestine 4* and *Lung 11*.

experiencing allergies or sinus congestion in the early morning, it may mean your Lungs need some extra attention. Luckily, there are several ways to keep them working smoothly.

Since the Lungs help to create Qi, exercise is very important. That's why I always make time for it in the morning. Just as many of my countrymen flock to the city parks at dawn to practice Qigong, I use this time of day to strengthen my Lung Qi while it's at its peak.

Tomorrow, instead of jumping out of bed late, gulping down some coffee, and rushing out the door, get up a little earlier. Massage your hands, head, and feet. Go outside and breathe the morning air. Even if you don't have time to jog or walk, do a few deep bends and stretches. Throw in a quick finger massage targeting the Lung meridian, specifically acupoints *Large Intestine 4* and *Lung 11* located on the fleshy part of your thumb root (see figure 7-2). Another good idea is to pause periodically throughout the day and take a few deep breaths, a habit that will keep your Lung energy moving.

Early Morning: Colon

As the morning progresses, you move toward the most active, Yang part of the day. The body is rested, the organs are strong, and you are now ready to energize your power centers.

The early hours between **5:00 and 7:00 a.m.** mark the time when the **Colon** is most active. It's when all of your digestive organs are operating at peak efficiency, producing Blood and Qi, vital fuel for the day.

Yet most people are unaware of this. They wake up in the morning and immediately launch into a multitude of activities—breakfast, kids, work, laundry—there's always so much to do. Few ever step back and think twice about those personal morning rituals that everyone shares.

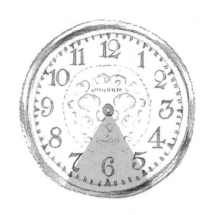

Bowel habits, for instance. Are you regular? Are your stools hard or dry? It may seem like a strange

5:00 to 7:00 a.m.—Colon

thing to evaluate, but for a Chinese doctor, everything connected to the body is important. A dry stool means that you may have too much Heat in the body. Chronic loose stools indicate there is too much Dampness. Both are symptoms that point to a Colon that needs some fine-tuning. This means starting each morning with a regular bowel movement, so that the Colon is empty and free to do its job for the rest of the day.

Many Colon issues are due to a poor diet and sedentary lifestyle. Instead of stocking up on dairy and sugary processed foods, why not reach for the roughage and fiber your digestive system thrives on? Again, be sure to move and breathe. This ensures that your digestive power plant efficiently delivers waste to the Colon. A good example of some colon-healthy foods are carrots; dark, leafy greens; and asparagus.

Morning: Spleen and Stomach

Do you generally skip breakfast and grab an "energy" bar on the commute to work? Or do you forget about eating altogether and

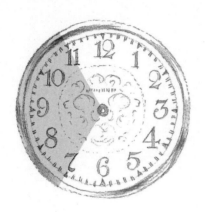

7:00 to 11:00 a.m. — Spleen and Stomach

catch up at lunch? From **7:00 to 11:00 a.m.** is the best time for your digestive organs to create the energy you will need for the rest of the day—but it can't happen unless you supply the raw material.

I often see people who don't have an appetite in the morning and can barely get down a glass of orange juice. Some become nauseated at the thought of a warm egg or a piece of toast. As I always tell these patients, "If your tank is empty, your engine can't run." Lacking the desire to eat in the morning is a sign you aren't properly feeding your kingdom.

Another sign is a lack of focus. The Spleen and Stomach don't just sort and process your food; they are also in charge of digesting your thoughts and processing information. If you find yourself fuzzy headed and unfocused in the morning, dependent on that jolt of caffeine to kick-start your energy, it might be that the digestive power players you depend on need some nourishing and strengthening.

STRENGTHEN YOUR SPLEEN

Tap the bottom of your rib cage ten times. This is acupressure point *Spleen 16.*

For most people I recommend a hearty breakfast with plenty of warm foods. Remember, cold foods such as yogurt and icy juice make your digestive organs work that much harder to transform the nutrients you need. A good breakfast should be warm, and include a mixture of protein, carbohydrates, and fruit.

Midday: Heart and Small Intestine

Noon marks the most powerful time of the day, what we call *Peak Yang*. Between **11 a.m. to 1:00 p.m.** and **1:00 to 3:00 p.m.** your **Heart** and its partner, the **Small Intestine**, are functioning at their optimum level. That's when your mind should be at its sharpest, your thought patterns their strongest, and your memory crystal clear.

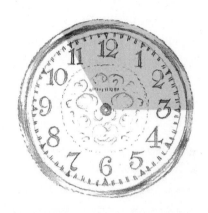

11:00 a.m. to 3:00 p.m.—Heart and Small Intestine

But as anyone who has nodded off in an early afternoon meeting can attest, often this is not the case.

Ask yourself: Do you tend to crash around noon? Does your mind get scattered? Are you forgetful? Maybe you're overly nervous or talkative at this time. All of this can mean your Heart network isn't getting the nourishment it needs. It is no wonder, then, that most heart attacks statistically happen around midday.

Should you find yourself experiencing palpitations, excessive perspiration, or shortness of breath around midday, it could be a warning sign that your Heart's meridians and Qi are imbalanced or blocked.

Because the Heart is strongest at noon, all the other organs of your body are benefiting as well, especially digestive organs such as the Small Intestine. The extra energy they are receiving powers them up to accept the noon meal and break it down into the nutritious Qi that you need.

This is why a warm, substantial lunch works so well. It's a critical part of your energy income, and important to eat every day. Beware of loading up on too many cold foods such as salads, sandwiches, and fruit shakes. At my clinic, we try to vary the flavor and temperature of our lunches. A typical meal might consist of marinated cucumber, beef or ham hock soup, along with a side of rice, and green tea.

Your digestive organs aren't the only beneficiaries of all that Heart energy. It is also flowing to other destinations around the body; your muscles and Lungs, for instance. This is a good time of day to take a break and go outside. If you can, fit in a walk or an easy jog. And always remember to fortify your body with fluids and nutrients afterward, so that you pay back your energy bank account.

Finally, it's important to balance any vigorous activity with a bit of rest. If you find yourself with ten minutes at the end of your lunch break, squeeze in a short nap. It all starts with managing your day and giving your power centers the right amount of food, exercise, and rest.

Afternoon: Kidneys and Bladder

In the afternoon your Yang energy begins its transition to Yin energy. From **3:00 to 7:00 p.m.** your **Kidneys** and **Bladder** are at their most active. Since the Kidneys are in charge of willpower and drive, this is one of the best times of the day to work on projects and get chores done.

If you lack the energy to finish an afternoon task or meet a project deadline, it means your Kidneys aren't putting out the power they should.

As the sun sets in the late afternoon you are halfway to Peak Yin.
At this time of day, who hasn't experienced chronic weariness and
the occasional cranky mood.
Maybe your lower back is painful,
you feel dizzy, or you frequently
feel the need to urinate. If these
clues ring a bell, it may be a sign
that your Kidneys are Deficient.

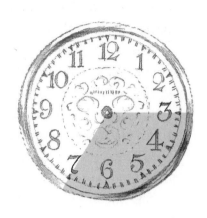

3:00 to 7:00 p.m.—Kidneys and
Bladder

Unfortunately, when people
experience these signs, they often
head right to the kitchen for a soda
or a salty bag of chips. They get that familiar but temporary boost of
Qi, but a few minutes later their Kidneys crash, and they flop on the
couch exhausted. The way to avoid this is to keep these organs
strong and balanced.

To avoid this, try these easy tips to keep that vital energy flowing
all afternoon: When feeling tired or energy deficient, stand up and
form your hands into loose fists. Place your right fist on the back of
your right hip and give it a good thump. Now, alternate by thumping
your left fist on your left hip. Take both fists and travel up the spinal
cord as high as you can go. By doing this exercise you are moving the
Qi in and around your Kidney meridians, delivering a refreshing
burst of energy. Or, if you like, you can try an EFT acupressure sequence by tapping on *all* of your power centers, and get even greater
results (see figure 5-4).

As I've mentioned, protein takes longer to digest than do simple
or processed carbohydrates such as sugar and flour products, giving
you a longer, more sustained energy boost. When a patient feels

constantly drained and exhausted, I often recommend a tablespoon-ful of protein powder in some milk or juice as a quick pick-me-up.

Snacks such as dates or nuts, sardines and crackers, or even some fruit with a bit of cheese are strengthening foods that are easily di-gestible, giving you added power during the late afternoon. This should work whether you are concentrating at the computer, per-forming physical labor, or studying. In every case, you are expending energy that needs to be replenished. A healthy protein snack will get you through the day a lot more readily than will a cup of coffee.

With your Kidneys providing powerful fuel, the afternoon is ex-cellent for getting your power centers moving. If you generally exer-cise at the end of the day, be sure to stretch out after a long day of sitting. Start slowly, with plenty of warm-up.

Evening: Triple Heater and Pericardium

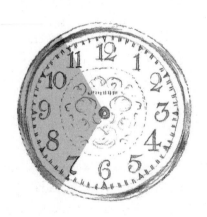

7:00 to 11:00 p.m.—Triple Heater/Pericardium

Now that the sun has set, your body begins its natural transition into the rest cycle. The period be-tween **7:00 and 11:00 p.m.** marks the dominance of two organs re-lated to the Heart: the **Triple Heater** and **Pericardium**. West-ern doctors do not recognize these organs and their meridians, but in Chinese medicine each plays an important part at this time of day.

The Triple Heater controls chemical processing and temperature in the upper, middle, and lower parts of your body. It also manages respiration and the nervous system, and that means it should remain healthy at all times of the day. The same is true for the Pericardium. This organ is a slippery membrane that protects the Heart, cushioning it from stress and shock. As with the Triple Heater, evening is when it is most sensitive.

As the day's Yang energy decreases, nature moves the body into a more restful Yin state (see figure 7-1). It's a transition your health depends on, a chance for the Heart and these other organs to get the much-needed break they deserve. But many people don't take heed.

Anyone who has lived in a big city has driven by the 24-hour gym and seen the treadmills humming with busy people determined to squeeze in their daily workout. This may *seem* like a good idea, but, in fact, pedaling furiously in the dead of night actually works against nature.

Why? From the Chinese perspective, these people are keeping their body in an active Yang state during the natural Yin time of day. The Heart and its related power centers are being forced to work their hardest *after* a stressful day of work. No wonder so many people have trouble with digestion and insomnia.

If kept up over time, a person's organs will become overtaxed, losing the ability to function the way they should. Soon, even more fuel will be required to keep their power plant running, depleting the very Qi they were hoping to gain at the gym.

To avoid this spiral, tailor your activities to the right time of day. In the evenings, wind down early and bring your body into a peaceful, restful state. Eat a lighter meal, and shift heavy workouts to other times of the day. An easy walk after dinner is healthy, but if you want a half-hour run, get up early and do it in the morning. And give your digestive organs some time off at night. Instead of a heavy four-course meal, think light—a soup or a warm sandwich, with some vegetables or fruit.

According to your body clock, morning is the best time for your digestive organs to do their job. That is why I recommend eating your heaviest meal of the day at midday. I have done so for most of my life and it has served me well.

A schedule like this is also a good idea for families. Nowadays school and office cafeterias serve large hot lunches. Take advantage, and eat your primary meal at midday, leaving the lighter foods for dinnertime. Not only is this beneficial to your system, it's another good way to lose weight.

Now that you're eating lighter, try having that evening meal three to four hours before bedtime. Eating right up until lights-out causes your digestive organs to kick into high gear during Yin rest time. The body's processing plant goes into overtime and soon you're tossing and turning, unable to sleep. Inevitably, the next day, there will be a fight to stay awake.

Another good idea is to avoid cold food, icy drinks, and caffeine before and at bedtime. The energy your body uses for heating cold foods puts a strain on the digestive system. Even some warm drinks are counterproductive. The extra Yang energy created by a late-night espresso surges through your meridians, making your restful Yin sleep state difficult to achieve. Spicy or greasy foods, especially if eaten regularly, are another road to sleepless nights.

Night: Liver and Gall Bladder

When **11:00 p.m.** rolls around, are you the type of person who feels like the day is just beginning? Maybe this is when you start firing off e-mails, calling friends, or vacuuming the house. Or maybe during late hours you suffer from chronic symptoms such as migraines and muscle cramps. These are all signs that the Liver and Gall Bladder are dominating your body's Qi cycle.

Between **11:00 p.m. to 1:00
a.m.** and **1:00 to 3:00 a.m.** these
power centers are at their most active. The Liver in particular, as the
commander of your body, is re-
plenishing and storing Blood before distributing it to the power
centers at a calm, even pace. All
the while, its companion organ,
the Gall Bladder, is storing and secreting bile produced by the Liver,
sending it off to the intestines in
order to help with digestion.

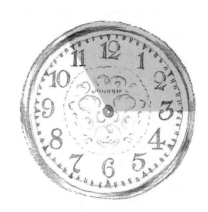

11:00 to 3:00 p.m.—Liver and Gall
Bladder

Because these organs are also responsible for the ability to make
decisions as well as maintaining flexible judgment, you must ensure
they aren't overtaxed in the middle of the night.

A sleepless night can make anyone angry, impulsive, and sometimes unable to make rational decisions. That's the Liver–Gall Bladder team announcing they haven't gotten the rest and relaxation they
require.

Other organs, such as the Heart, also play a part in calming you
during this time of night (see chapter 2). For all these power centers to
do their jobs properly, the Yang energy of the day needs an opportunity to fully transition into the Yin of the evening and nighttime hours.

When this transition doesn't occur, it creates a disharmony between Yin and Yang. This usually happens when the day's work continues into the evening, or strong emotions can't be put aside.
Sometimes it's as simple as eating a late-night bean burrito.

The good news is that keeping the Liver and Gall Bladder balanced doesn't have to be difficult. As the day dwindles into evening,
relax and slow down. Move from Yang to Yin activities. Save exercise,

studying, or physical work for earlier in the day. Taking some time to read and relax will help you ease into to a Yin state more readily.

An effective technique is to visualize yourself in a calm, restful place, then begin to systematically relax the muscles in each part of your body. This sends signals that you are ready to shut down and lets your power centers operate in their most efficient manners to do their jobs.

Sometimes a short meditation, even just voicing a "thank you" before sleep, eases me into rest. A few of my patients will add a few drops of lavender and chamomile to water and use it to spray the bedroom when they feel particularly wired.

If you find yourself agitated or uncomfortable during the night, try soothing some relevant pressure points. Rub your big toe and the indentation between the big toe and the second toe (figure 3-8). This point marks the beginning of the Liver meridian. You can also massage your shoulders and the back of your head, which houses your Gall Bladder meridian. If tapping acupressure points (figure 5-4) works for you, try an EFT sequence that releases built-up worries.

By making yourself aware of how and when your daily Qi is flowing, you can use these tools to better manage and deflect health issues when they arise.

MARIANNE JAS'S STORY: SCHEDULING MY BODY CLOCK

If I have learned anything from my illness, it is the fundamental role my body clock plays in keeping me healthy.

Before becoming sick, I was never a morning person. Waking up was a chore, and when I finally did crawl out of bed, I was unfocused and muzzy-headed for hours. Instead of breakfast, I usually had two cups of java and a sweet roll before I resembled a functioning human being.

I know now that my fatigue, lack of concentration, and need for sugary stimulants were due to a weak Stomach and Spleen network. It was a risky state to be in because I didn't have enough Blood and Qi to go around, affecting my body's other functions.

Once Esther's acupuncture and herbal treatments began, I added the healthy breakfasts I had been missing. I also stopped skipping the other meals my body was craving. My concentration increased and so did my morning energy reserves.

Each day now starts with a 6:30 a.m. wakeup call, followed either by exercise (walking two to three miles) or brief meditation.

Other habits have changed as well. In my old life I used to stuff down a lunchtime sub or a few protein bars at the computer. Nowadays I make an effort to get up and take a physical break away from my workspace. At midday, it's usually a hot meal, if possible followed by a 10- to 15-minute catnap if possible.

Another good idea is to prepare meals using a slow cooker. They're useful for creating a variety of simple meals ahead of time, and they also allow the use of cheaper cuts of meat and fish, not only saving money but delivering delicious results as well.

Esther offered me one more important piece of advice. In the past I tended to work straight through the evening. This seemed normal to me, but Esther warned me that the excessive concentration was affecting my Stomach and Spleen's ability to process Blood and Qi. Now I stop work in the early evening and make sure I eat a light supper. This gives me time to wind down at least two hours before bedtime, and my organs have the time they need to slow down and relax. My husband is a lot happier, and best of all, I find I'm more rested and ready for sleep.

Adjusting meals, work, and rest according to my body's energy needs was a revelation. By paying attention to my internal clock I was able to give my power centers exactly what they needed, when they needed it. Now, when I feel that familiar exhausted feeling, I stop, take stock of my schedule, and make the adjustments I know will put my energy on the right track.

The Rhythm of the Seasons

Just as Blood and Qi rises and falls with the 24-hour cycle of sun and moon, humans also are affected by a much larger, universal cycle: the earth's vast journey around the sun.

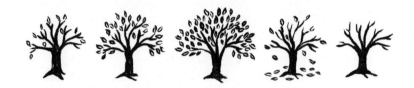

Not only are our power centers synchronized with the *daily* rise and fall of the sun and moon, they are also synchronized to the *annual* cycle of the seasons (see figure 7-3).

Summer, of course, has the longest days. It's the warmest season and the time when Blood and Qi pump the fastest. During the colder, darker months of winter, Qi contracts and moves inward, conserving energy and keeping the body warm.

Understanding how your power centers are affected by the seasons makes it possible to maximize your energy throughout the year.

Spring

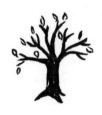

Strange though it may seem, spring is the first season of the Chinese calendar year. It's a time of powerful Yang energy, new growth, and renewal. In spring the earth begins moving closer to the sun and the days stretch out.

This is the time of year when the energy of the earth is lifted and it is time to rid ourselves of winter's stagnation. But weather can be unstable at this time of year. As the shoulder season between winter and summer, spring often gives us rain and dampness that can make it difficult to stay warm and dry.

In this season, I ask my patients not to let the warmer weather fool them into dressing for summer. By wearing tank tops and shorts, they are exposing their meridians to an invasion of Cold and Wind.

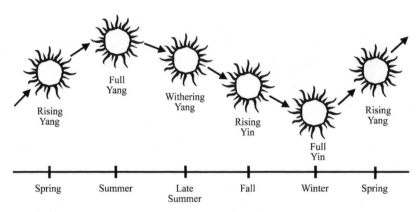

7-3. Seasonal Yin and Yang Cycle

And, as everyone knows, a nasty spring flu can be uncomfortable and inconvenient.

Spring is also when the Liver and Gall Bladder, the strategists of the body, are most sensitive. They need to be supported with the right foods and proper exercise.

Eat more complex carbohydrates, such as whole grains, and dark, leafy greens such as kale, mustard, and chard. Since warmer foods only create heat and stress, stay away from too much caffeine, alcohol, sugar and fatty, spicy foods. Instead of reaching for sodas and coffee, drink water with lemon to clear Liver heat and stabilize digestion.

EAT GREEN, THE COLOR OF SPRING

Collards	Green onions
Spinach	Kale
Mustard greens	Chard
Green apples	

Spring is also a wonderful time to exercise, especially if you have been less active during the winter months. Stagnation causes blockages that result in muscle tension, digestive disturbances, allergies, irritability, and depression.

Finally, to make the most out of this powerful season of growth, go to bed early and rise a little earlier than usual.

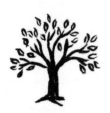

Summer

Moving past spring and its rising Yang energy, we reach summer, the season of *full* Yang (see Figure 7-3). The earth is closest to the sun and temperatures are at their peak. Qi and Blood are flowing with strength and power, making this the perfect time to stretch yourself physically and mentally.

It's also the best time of year to spend outdoors. Daylight lasts longer, so naturally you should want to be more active—exercising, socializing, working in the yard. But with all this activity, keeping your body cool will pay dividends. Too much perspiration dries out the body, making it even more important to drink well and keep those internal fluids circulating.

With the rise in summer heat, the Heart in particular is sensitive to changes in temperature. If the summer months are making you feel exhausted or mentally disoriented, protect your energy bank account by giving your king plenty of rest.

If you are experiencing palpitations or shortness of breath, or find yourself overly jumpy and nervous, it could indicate that too much activity during this time of year has put a strain on the Heart and its meridians. Other symptoms you might experience include fevers, dehydration, and heat rashes. If you recognize these symptoms (see page 8) a Chinese doctor might be able to help. One of the best ways to nourish and strengthen this organ is with food and diet.

On the hottest days, I recommend cooling foods that will lower your body temperature: seasonal produce such as salad, fruit, tofu, cucumber, or some Mung Bean Soup (see page 34). Try an apple or a few pieces of watermelon, or drink some natural lemonade sweetened with maple syrup, honey, or agave nectar.

EAT RED, THE COLOR OF SUMMER

Tomato	Raspberries
Apple	Strawberries
Cherries	Watermelon

Summer is also a good time to fire up the barbecue and lightly grill or sauté small amounts of fish and meats. If your system runs Cold, cut down on raw foods and cooling drinks. Instead, cook those vegetables with meat if you prefer, and add warming spices, such as ginger or cinnamon.

To satisfy your parched throat, try brewing up some mint or chamomile tea. But stay away from greasy and heavily fried foods. Hot weather is not the time to make your Heart, Liver, and Spleen work overtime.

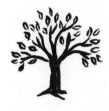

Late Summer

As summer winds down and the days get cooler and shorter, every part of nature is affected by the coming change of season, and the human body is no exception.

The months of late August to early September are considered the middle point of the Chinese calendar year. As the earth tilts away from the sun, the Yang of summer is transitioning to the Yin of fall to come.

This is the time of year when the Spleen and Stomach are most at the mercy of weather and seasonal changes.

If you are experiencing bloating, indigestion, weight gain, or nausea during this time of year, it's important to pay extra attention to what you eat.

When confronted with summer heat it's common to gravitate toward cooling foods and drinks, which is mostly a good thing. But that enticing ice-cold double ice cream shake has a lot of mucus-forming dairy and sugar, and may have the opposite effect. Remember that the dairy-sugar combination actually heats up your digestive organs, creating a damp, Phlegm-like substance (Tan) that blocks their function.

As discussed in previous chapters, this dampness can lead to stomach discomfort and weight gain. When your body has to heat foods straight from the freezer, it takes a lot of energy it needs for other things. Digestion in particular slows to a sluggish pace, leading to that unwelcome combination of bloating and gas.

As we transition into fall, a smooth dietary transition starts with easing from summer's colder, raw foods and moving to warmer choices that help your body get ready for winter.

EAT YELLOW, THE COLOR OF LATE SUMMER

Squash	Garbanzo beans
Corn	Sweet potatoes
Yukon gold potatoes	Sweet rice
Lemons	

Try preparing meals made from yellow: squash, corn, sweet potatoes, millet, potatoes, and sweet rice with a sprinkle of saffron. All these natural ingredients strengthen the Blood and balance the digestion, giving your body exactly what it needs to prepare for the colder seasons to come.

Fall

As fall takes hold, the earth begins its annual rotation away from the sun. The green foliage of summer withers and the air turns cold, windy, and dry. It's a natural process of conserving energy, a chance to build for the winter months. People, too, follow this natural cycle, making this the perfect time to wind down and cut back on intense activity.

I can still see myself as a small girl stepping outside our clinic on West Nanjing Street. In early October a cold breeze would sweep in off the ocean and my mother would wrap us in coats and tell us to keep our Wei Qi (immune system) protected. Later, when I studied medicine, I understood why she was so adamant. As the air temperature drops, one's Qi turns inward, slowing and contracting, making it easier for the Five Devils to take hold.

Fall is an especially delicate time for your Qi leader, the Lungs. Every time you take a breath on a brisk evening, you are inhaling cool, dry air. This is generally not harmful; but become fatigued or overly emotional, and Wei Qi weakens, making it easy for a bronchial virus or flu to attack the Lungs.

Several herbal formulas are helpful during the fall flu season. Gan Mao Ling Tea and Yin Chiao Jie Du Wan (Honeysuckle and Forsythia Clear Toxins Pills) are two choices your Chinese practitioner might suggest. They are available over the counter at designated herbal and health food stores.

EAT WHITE, THE COLOR OF FALL

Pears	Potato
Cauliflower	Daikon radish

Remember that the Lungs actually work closely with their partner organ, the Colon (see page 5). Dry skin and dry stools are a sure sign that this organ is weak and needs attention.

Many of my patients have trouble staying healthy during this in-between time of year. Often, days are still warm, fooling them into forgetting a coat for those cooler evenings. There is less sunlight, causing them to sacrifice the exercise and movement vital to keeping illnesses at bay. And when it's cooler outside, many forgo the deep breathing that is so necessary to creating Qi and Blood.

This is why it's so important to adjust your habits to fit the season. Yes, it seems obvious, but dress warmly. Go to bed a little earlier than you did during the summer months, and do some calming exercises before bed.

When it's time to eat, choose foods that strengthen, nourish, and support the Lungs: Almonds and dried apricots will build strength, as will winter squash and root vegetables. Turnips and foods from the onion family are good because they create warmth and heat. If you are suffering from dry skin or stools, try adding some ingredients that moisturize, such as mushrooms, pears, and honey (see page 101).

SOOTHING PEAR SKIN TEA FOR THE LUNGS

YIELD: 1 CUP

INGREDIENTS:
1 PEAR
1 CUP WATER
HONEY

Peel the pear, saving the skin. Place the pear skin in the 1 cup of water and boil for approximately 20 minutes. Remove and discard the skin, add honey to taste, and drink throughout the day.

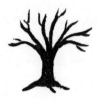

Winter

When the winter months roll around, the earth is farthest from the sun, a time known as Full Yin (see figure 7-3). Lung Qi is taking a backseat, and now the Kidneys and their sister organ, the Bladder, are in charge.

The Kidneys are your ministry of power, so if you overextend yourself during the summer months, it's possible to experience a drop in energy during the winter. If you feel cold and exhausted, for instance, your energy account needs to be replenished. This will be evident with signs of Deficiency: Pale skin, dark circles under the eyes, night sweats, and insomnia. All are warnings from the Kidneys that your power supply is running low.

This is why winter is a good time to conserve and replenish Qi, Blood, and Jing. Go to bed as early as you can, and rise a bit later than usual. If the shortage of sunlight affects you, or if you are chronically depressed and fearful during this time of year, you can keep your Qi flowing by tapping or rubbing along the Kidney and Bladder meridians. And if the sun is peeking out, just ten minutes outside can bring some much-needed Yang energy into your life.

Also, pay particular attention to dressing for the weather. The Kidneys reside in the lower back, so a bare midriff in an icy wind only makes it easier for the Cold Devil to invade. An attack like this on the Kidneys and Bladder energy pathways can result in everything from a sore back to menstrual pains or a major bout of flu.

If you're experiencing exhaustion during the winter months, take care to limit exercise in the snow and cold. Consider joining an indoor gym or yoga studio. You could also ask your practitioner about a helpful herbal formula called Lieu Wei Di Huang Wan (Six Gentlemen Tea Pills), which helps to strengthen the Kidneys.

The cold season is the best time to eat foods that create energy and warm your body. Hearty soups, stews, whole grains, and nuts are all great foods that aid digestion during this natural slowdown.

If you love bitter black coffee and double-salted pretzels, indulge yourself a bit during these months. Surprisingly, the Kidneys can actually benefit from a moderate portion of salty and bitter foods.

Other foods beneficial to the Kidneys in wintertime include protein-rich, warming foods such as lamb, beef, dates, lotus seeds, soy sauce, ginseng, ginger, and cinnamon. If your body is running cold, even a little wine can boost the circulation and create warmth. Other healthy winter dishes include hearty soups and broths and whole grains.

EAT BLUE-BLACK, THE COLOR OF WINTER

Dates   Black beans
Plums   Black sesame seeds
Eggplant

By eating right in the winter season, you are preparing your body for the next cycle to resume again in spring.

Follow Nature's Rhythms

Like every living thing, human beings are intricately connected to the ageless cycle of sun and moon; of light and darkness. If you pay attention, this cycle will tell you when to work and when to rest, when to eat and when to move. Synchronizing your daily activities to match these internal and external clocks is the best way to manage and protect the body's energy account.

The key lies with you and your ability to listen to your body. Whether there is a simple imbalance or a more serious illness, your power centers will show warning signs. They can come at a certain time of day or a certain season. All you have to know is where and when to look.

Fainting spells and disturbed speech at noon or during the summer can mean your Heart needs to be cooled off.

Tinnitus or achy bones and knees in the late afternoon are often a sign of weak Kidneys and Bladder.

A painful muscle spasm or migraine in the middle of the night might be your Liver needing attention.

Once you begin to understand and release the anxiety these symptoms generate, I assure you the intensity of the physical problems can be greatly minimized. My patients always tell me that once they understand that the Liver is generating painful migraines in the middle of the night, they remain calm and take the proper steps to find relief.

In the long run, it is the proper combination of food, exercise, visualization, and treatment will bring that organ back in balance. Often, symptoms can miraculously disappear with a small dose of self-applied treatment.

It's not necessary to adhere to a rigid set of rules about sunrise, weather, and season. The important thing is to aim for a healthy balance that moves you through each day with ease and grace.

Using these natural rhythms in my own life, I have overcome illness, built a busy medical practice, and maintained the energy to take care of my family. I credit all of this to following nature's cycles, a simple practice that I am positive will also work for you.

DR. TING'S TOTAL HEALTH ESSENTIALS

DAILY CLOCK
Sunrise: Rising Yang
Noon: Peak Yang
Sunset: Rising Yin
Midnight: Peak Yin

BODY CLOCK

Lungs	**Bladder**
3:00 to 5:00 a.m.	3:00 to 5:00 p.m.
Colon	**Kidneys**
5:00 to 7:00 a.m.	5:00 to 7:00 p.m.
Spleen	**Pericardium**
7:00 to 9:00 a.m.	7:00 to 9:00 p.m.
Stomach	**Triple Heater**
9:00 to 11:00 a.m.	9:00 to 11:00 p.m.
Heart	**Gall Bladder**
11:00 a.m. to 1:00 p.m.	11:00 p.m. to 1:00 a.m.
Small Intestine	**Liver**
1:00 to 3:00 p.m.	1:00 to 3:00 a.m.

ORGANS AND THE SEASONS

Spring: Liver and Gall Bladder
Summer: Heart and Small Intestine
Late Summer: Spleen and Stomach
Fall: Lungs and Colon
Winter: Kidneys and Bladder

8

Clear Out the Blockages
Healing Techniques and Treatments

For as long as I can remember I have always wanted to be a doctor. From an early age I followed my parents and their students on hospital rounds. I couldn't wait to run next door and fetch patient prescriptions from the pharmacy, rich with the smells of exotic herbs and powders. After finishing my homework, I would even memorize acupressure points from medical texts.

One morning, my knowledge was tested firsthand. I was eating breakfast when my sister Rhoda stumbled in. She was clutching her jaw in intense pain and was unable to speak. I wasn't sure what was wrong, but with my parents away seeing patients, there was no one else to help. I grabbed an acupuncture needle and placed it directly on her jawbone at a place I hoped was *Stomach 7*—a point along the Stomach meridian that controls the jaw. Rhoda let out a loud scream. Had I failed? After a few anxious seconds, Rhoda's jaw relaxed. She began talking—a little bit at first, then a mile a minute in her usual way. I had done it!

For me it was a turning point. If I could help someone with a needle and a little knowledge, what could I do as a fully trained doctor?

Years later I often feel like an experienced sea captain, on the lookout for everything from a flulike squall to a life-threatening typhoon. Often these storms may not manifest themselves for years to come, but the signs are always there. The symptoms can be emotional or physical, but with careful analysis they give me all the clues I need to steer your body to a safe harbor.

A Doctor's Role: Considering the Whole

For many, the decision to visit a Chinese practitioner can be full of apprehension: What will it be like? . . . Is acupuncture painful? . . . Will other exotic treatments be used? In nearly every case my patients find their visit a positive experience.

Unlike Western medicine, which tends to focus on individual symptoms, Chinese medicine is interested in the whole person. I consider each aspect of my patients' life: Family issues, working conditions, and lifestyle habits. Even current weather patterns can provide me with critical clues to what might be wrong. This tends to give people confidence that I am looking at their problem from a total body perspective. But the differences go even further.

Whereas Western doctors often prescribe medicines to target and suppress external symptoms, Chinese doctors choose to treat the *root cause* of the problem. To understand why, let's look at the way your energy system works and what you'll experience when a Chinese doctor diagnoses and treats your health problem.

A Doctor's Role: Balancing Yin and Yang

All illness stems from a basic imbalance of overall energy, between your Yin and your Yang. When you are healthy, these two mutually opposed energies live in an evenly balanced state. But when they tilt out of equilibrium, it becomes the job of a Chinese physician to find out why.

Yin is a cold, passive, and serene energy. It's what you feel when you're calm and relaxed. Yang is an active, fiery energy, signifying movement, excitement, anger, and thrills. To maintain good health, both must coexist peacefully and in equal measure within your body-kingdom. For many people, this balance can be challenging to achieve.

How can I tell whether your Yin and Yang energies are balanced? If your overall Yin energy is too strong, you may chill easily. If, however, your Yang energy is too dominant, you might experience a fever, or too much Heat. In either case, a Chinese practitioner can bring these two energies back into balance with acupuncture and herbs.

When considering healing from this perspective, it's easy to see that the physical body is just the visible outer portion of a complex web of energy. This life force, or Qi, flows within you and is the very first thing I evaluate when treating a patient.

I access this energy circuitry by a few simple means—some may seem exotic at first, but they have been proven effective for thousands of years.

Tools of the Trade: Acupuncture

Acupuncture was discovered more than three thousand years ago. It was first introduced in print within the pages of the *Nei Jing*, the Yellow Emperor's Classic, in AD 200.

Acupuncture grew and developed over centuries through meticulous study and analysis. Ancient Chinese doctors systematically inserted needles into specific points and observed the effects on various

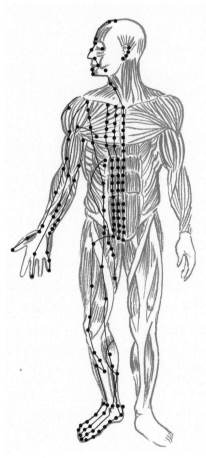

Acupuncture Points and Meridians

parts of the body. The results led them to map and record an intricate system of channels.

The main goals of acupuncture are to manipulate, activate, and move the flow of Qi through these meridians by needling points, or "gateways," along the energy channels. There are approximately 365 acupuncture points on the surface of fourteen energy channels running throughout your body. An intricate system indeed!

No wonder Chinese physicians receive years of schooling to determine precisely which points will be most beneficial for a patient's specific imbalance.

Of course, in the intervening three thousand years, acupuncture has seen many significant advances. In ancient times the needles were made from materials at hand, such as flint, bone, and silver. Today our disposable needles are made from steel, in sizes ranging from half an inch to five inches in length. These needles are so tiny that most people never feel when they're inserted.

The length and width of each needle varies depending on the area being worked on. For example, a practitioner will use a thicker needle for a fleshy part of the body such as the buttocks, and a thinner needle for the slim layer of skin on the scalp. There are also spe-

cialized tools called "press" needles for
working with certain points on the ear.

What to Expect from
Acupuncture

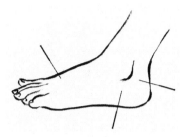

Typically, an acupuncture treatment involves the use of twelve to fifteen needles placed along specific meridians. A
session usually consists of one or more

Acupuncture needles are made of
steel, ranging from half an inch to
five inches in length.

rounds of needles, which are left in from twenty minutes to whatever
time the acupuncturist feels is necessary.

Like any procedure, acupuncture is a highly personal experience,
and everyone reacts differently. Although many of my patients do not
feel a thing when I insert a needle, some may feel some minor discomfort. Reactions during and after the treatment range from a sleepy
feeling to becoming highly energized. Others feel nothing at all.

It's important to note that "feeling" a sensation is not necessarily
an indicator of how well the treatment is working. Improvements in
your health condition are dependent on numerous factors: the
unique nature of the specific symptoms, how your body responds to
treatment, and the number
of treatments you undergo.

Everyone wants instant
results, and often, acupuncture *can* offer immediate relief. Other times, the results
take a while. Keep in mind
that acupuncture heals by
changing the *flow* of energy
or Qi, and that means the
body needs time to adjust.

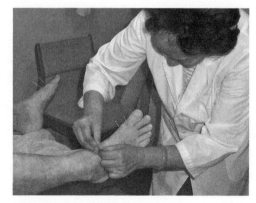

Esther doing acupuncture

Other Forms of Treatment

Moxibustion

Moxibustion refers to the use of burned, dried mugwort that is applied directly to the skin or above certain acupuncture points. Its effectiveness lies in reaching the meridians with penetrating Heat, thus moving and circulating Stagnant masses of Blood and Qi. Commonly called *moxa*, the substance is applied in the form of a cigarlike tube, much like a small cigar; and when lit it gives off a smoky, musky odor. Moxa can also be burned in a box placed on the body so that Heat is dispersed over a larger area.

Moxibustion is generally used when someone is in a Deficient or weakened condition, to energize and stimulate organ function. It definitely should *not* be used if a person is suffering from inner Heat or is pregnant. It is best to visit a practitioner first before applying moxibustion.

Chinese Massage (Tui Na)

If you've ever gone to a spa and the masseuse has made your day, you can thank *Tui Na* (Chinese massage). Dating back to 2700 BC, Tui Na

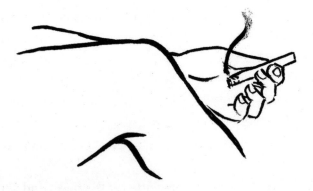

Figure 8-1. Treating with moxa can alleviate symptoms.

is one of the primary methods Chinese physicians use to treat illness, and is the forefather to all modern massage and bodywork. If you find acupuncture needles intimidating, Tui Na can be a great substitute or sister therapy. It works by having the doctor manually manipulate various points and meridians, using his or her hands, elbows, and fingers to stimulate and move your Blood and Qi.

Before treating patients by this method, the Tui Na practitioner must be educated in many specific ailments as well as in musculoskeletal anatomy. A session typically consists of various rolling, kneading, grasping, and pressing techniques that put pressure on certain meridian points. The results are usually just as effective as acupuncture, and many people have found it to be a great help in healing a variety of stubborn conditions.

Herbal Formulas

I hear it every time a new patient walks into my office: "What is that interesting smell?" If you're not used to it, the pungent aroma of Chinese herbs can seem strange at first. Fortunately, most of my patients find it quite calming and pleasing.

Chinese herbal therapy goes back to the third century AD, and is one of the primary tools of a Chinese doctor. One of the foremost instructional manuals in the field, *Shang Han Luan* (Discussion of Cold-Induced Disorders), was published in AD 219, and many of its prescriptions and formulas are still used by clinics and hospitals all over the world.

Since the appearance of *Shang Han Luan*, thousands of books have been written documenting the clinical methods that many doctors—including my own great-grandfather—have used to heal their patients.

Herbs are very easy to take, gentle on the body, and generally have few side effects. When used alongside acupuncture to balance the Yin and Yang, they help to warm or cool, dry or moisten, energize or calm various blockages.

The word *herb* is actually a bit misleading, as the term actually goes beyond plants and refers to an entire range of organic substances, including minerals and even animal matter. Most herbal formulas contain a combination of these different substances. Here are some examples of typical ingredients categorized by their source material:

- **Minerals**—Shi Gao (gypsum)
- **Roots**—Bai Shao (white peony)
- **Leaves**—Ai Ye (mugwort)
- **Seeds**—Niu Bang Zhi (burdock)
- **Peels**—Chen Pi (tangerine)
- **Twigs**—Gui Zhi (cinnamon)

With over three hundred herbs to choose from, prescribing the right combination for a specific condition takes training and experience. I base my decision on the characteristics of each herb that best matches an individual's symptoms.

ANTIVIRAL/ANTIBACTERIAL HERBS

Antibacterial and antiviral herbs have been used in place of antibiotics for many centuries. Here are a few that have been proven to be highly effective.

Chai Hu (thorowax): antibacterial, antiviral, antimalarial; used for feverish colds, malaria

Ge Gen (kudzu vine): antispasmodic; used for chills, measles, dysentery

Huang Lian (Chinese Gold Thread): antibacterial; used for gastroenteritis, food poisoning, fevers, boils, abscesses

Huan Qin (baikal skullcap): antibacterial; used for chills, yellow sputum, dysentery, urinary tract infection

Jin Yin Hua (honeysuckle): antibacterial, antiviral; used for colds, fever caused by wind and heat, urinary tract infections, boils and abscesses

Ju Hua (chrysanthemum): antibacterial, antifungal; used for sore red eyes, dizziness, headaches

Lian Qiao (forsythia): antibacterial, antiparasitic; used for infections caused by abscess

Niu Bang Zhi (burdock): antibacterial, antifungal; used for throat inflammations, tonsillitis, mumps, measles, carbuncles

Some herbs contain animal parts, at times a controversial issue in the West. Remember that when these ingredients were first formulated many centuries ago, animals were a primary means of survival and sustenance. They were analyzed and various parts proven effective in healing disease. Oysters, abalone shells, and cuttlefish bones are prime examples of animals and animal parts that have proven to work in treating high blood pressure, insomnia, and nervous exhaustion.

Of course, I do not condone the illegal use of any animal product, endangered or otherwise, nor do I support the controversial practices some doctors in China and elsewhere still continue to use today. With all of the many plant- and mineral-based treatment options available, I recommend that you talk with your practitioner and make sure he or she meets acceptable standards of ethical care.

Individually, herbs have certain properties that affect your system. It is in combination with one another, however, that they reach their true potential.

I like to think of an herbal formula as a football team. When I prescribe a certain combination, my first and foremost goal is to activate and unblock Qi. My herbal team should burst through the blockage and get the Qi flowing smoothly, freeing the patient of pain and discomfort. It's a group effort, and each herb plays either an offensive or defensive role. Like any successful team, it takes carefully chosen players and a good coach to win. That's why it's important to trust a Chinese doctor to build the right combination of herbs for your specific health condition.

Temperature and Direction of Herbs

Herbs also work like a mini-thermometer. Each has a specific temperature—**Cold, Cool, Neutral, Hot**, and **Warm**—which needs to be matched to the problem being targeted.

For example, if someone complains of fever and an itchy rash, I'll choose a formula that *cools* and *moistens*. If a person suffers from a cold and lacks energy, I'll prescribe herbs that are *warm* and *energizing*. Infections have their own properties, so I'll blend an *antimicrobial* or *antiviral* herb to "kick" the virus out. I still remember one of my teachers, the great herbalist Dr. Zhang Ying, telling us to use herbs to "attack" illness with the same force and dexterity as a warrior wields his weapons.

In addition, herbs work in a certain *direction*. By carefully choosing formulas, we can send energy to the very areas that need it most. For a headache accompanied by rising heat and red eyes, I'll choose herbs that direct the energy *downward*. If a person is suffering from extreme fatigue, I'll choose a formula that directs energy *upward*, to stimulate and increase circulation.

How do we know what direction an herb travels? Just look at the way it grows in nature. Underground plants such as roots and tubers tend to work downward. That also goes for seeds, fruits, and minerals that fall to the ground. Upward-growing plants such as flowers and leaves tend to lift the energy or virus up and out.

As your body absorbs these herbs it begins to change and adapt, and that's why we occasionally need to adjust the formula. Western medicine often prescribes the same medication for at least ten days, whereas a Chinese herbalist will alter a prescription according to what your body is saying during each visit. The idea is not to heal the symptom but to clear the blockage and at the same time nourish, strengthen, and balance the body.

In each case the herbs are matched to the patient's condition, and when taken regularly for a number of weeks, they usually lead to a distinct improvement if not a complete turnaround. Sometimes the results can seem miraculous, as I have experienced in my own health.

HERBS AND TEMPERATURE

Cold herbs: Da Huang (Chinese rhubarb), Zhi Zi (Gardenia)

Slightly Cool herbs: Bai Shao (white peony), Bo He (field mint), Chai Hu (thorowax), Chi Shao (red peony)

Cool herbs: Ge Gen (kudzu vine), Xia Ku Cao (self-heal), Xi Yang Shen (American ginseng)

Neutral herbs: Fu Ling (China root), Gan Cao (licorice), Dang Shen (codonopsis), Gu Ya (rice)

Warm herbs: Dang Gui (Chinese angelica), Du Zhong (eucommia), Xio Hui Xiang (fennel)

Hot herbs: Bi Ba (Indian long pepper)

An Herbal Cure for Tuberculosis: Esther

One morning, when I was nineteen years old, I woke up severely nauseated. It hurt to breathe and I began to cough up blood. At first I thought it was a bad flu, but a few days later the lab tests confirmed I had tuberculosis.

Even at that age I knew how powerful Chinese herbs could be. My mother placed me on a daily regimen to strengthen my Lungs and clear the infection. I put all of my faith in the tools and the process, and in time my Lungs became toned and strong. Eventually, I was symptom free, and I entered medical school that next fall.

Acupuncturist vs. Herbalist

Not all acupuncturists are herbalists, and vice versa. If your Chinese practitioner also dispenses herbs, find out if he or she has passed the National Certification Commission's exam for Acupuncture and Oriental Medicine. Practitioners in California and Nevada require a special exam to be permitted to dispense Chinese herbs. In other states, herbal certification is voluntary, so make sure you are informed.

How to Take Chinese Herbs, Teas, Pills, and Powders

Traditionally, the most common way to take herbs is in their raw form. Many of my patients are bewildered when they're first handed a bagful of tree bark, roots, seeds, minerals, and tiny stones. I gently remind them that though herbs may appear different than other prescriptions they're used to, each ingredient has a role that is critical in clearing their illness and restoring their health.

The process starts when your practitioner creates an herbal mixture expressly for you. He or she will select the herbs, then weigh and divide them into appropriate doses. Each dose is then placed into an individual bag, which you take home, boil, and strain, before drinking the liquid.

The formula, or *Tang*, is boiled with water for thirty minutes, until it becomes a tea that is swallowed twice a day (see figure 8-2).

Patented Herbs: Pills and Capsules

Many classic Chinese herbal formulas are now manufactured for mass consumption. Powdered herbs, for instance, are a granulated version of raw herbs that can be added to water. This powder is

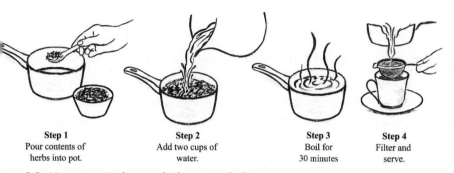

Step 1	**Step 2**	**Step 3**	**Step 4**
Pour contents of herbs into pot.	Add two cups of water.	Boil for 30 minutes	Filter and serve.

gure 8-2. Measuring, Boiling, and Filtering Herbal Tea

ground from a raw generic formula, then poured into capsules, or compressed into tablet form.

Patented herbs are another form of classical herbal formulas. Although these generic herbs are manufactured in China and exported to the West, a growing number of U.S. and European manufacturers are creating their own variations of these formulas.

Generic, patented herbs are usually prescribed for a certain group of patients who, for a variety of reasons, are unable to drink the powders or teas. For them, a tablet or pill is a good alternative to drinking a formula they can't stomach or have trouble digesting. These herbs are safe to take for extended periods of time.

I often prescribe these patented herbal formulas in my own practice. Although they can be purchased over the counter, it is best to consult with a Chinese doctor first. Generic formulas can be very effective, yet they are nonetheless drugs and have a specific purpose. The wrong herb can easily make a serious condition worse.

Herbs, acupuncture, and Tui Na are but some of the many tools in a Chinese doctor's arsenal. To use them in the most effective way, a patient should always see a physician for a proper diagnosis.

The Four Examinations

So you've made the decision to try a Chinese doctor. You walk in, a bit unsure, slightly scared maybe, but you're also ready. After trying a number of treatment options you just want to get better.

At first, a Chinese practitioner's office isn't what you might expect. Because a Chinese doctor relies mainly on observing intricate clues on and around the body, the office is generally quite simple: a desk, and two chairs situated a few feet from each other.

"My first visit to your office was somewhat startling," a former patient told me recently. "There were no machines, no scales, no EKG. You didn't even use a stethoscope. Yet your examination was incredibly thorough."

If you had visited Fuzhou Road, Shanghai, in 1916 you would have seen my great-grandfather, Dr. Ding Gangren, using nearly the same techniques and diagnosis. As founder of the first teaching college in China and the most celebrated practitioner of his day, he would wait until his patients sat down facing his large desk, then begin his intricate diagnosis. Like every generation of Chinese doctors before him he used the same four practices:

- Looking
- Listening and smelling
- Asking
- Touching

Today, every Chinese doctor uses exactly the same techniques. By following this process, I can discover a wealth of information just as my great-grandfather did. I begin with *looking* at your eyes, skin, and tongue, then *listening* to your voice and *smelling* body odors. After that I *ask* about symptoms and habits, and finally *touch* your wrist to take a pulse reading.

Although this process may be different from what you're used to, the end goal is the same—healing the body as quickly as possible.

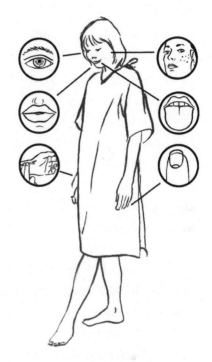

First Examination: Looking
Eyes

When I first observe patients, it's important to find out *where* their problem originated, and *what type* of problem it is. For this I get up close and personal, putting myself inches from their eyes.

This is the first place I look for a good reason. Within the eyes there are clues to the health of the entire body. Even the physical condition of a person's power centers can be read by looking carefully at his or her eyes.

First Examination: Looking

The eye is subdivided into seven sections, each revealing a little bit more about a patient's energy level and overall health (see figure 8-3). Consider some of these typical conditions:

• **Bright, clear, white eyes:** Normal
• **Red eyes:** Excessive Heat, Heart, Liver condition
• **Yellow eyes:** Dampness, Stomach and Spleen condition
• **Yellow discharge:** Infection
• **Watery eyes:** Infection, Kidney condition

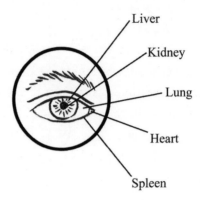

Figure 8-3. Map of the Eye

- **Rapid eye movements:** Nervous condition
- **Pupil:** Kidney condition
- **Floaters and blurry vision:** Energy Deficiency, Liver condition
- **Under-eye bags:** Spleen disharmony
- **Under-eye dark rings:** Kidney Deficiency

By analyzing these signs, I have a reliable source of information, a window into my patient's internal physical condition. Other clues, too, help complete this picture.

THE ROLE OF FLUIDS

Fluids refer to all the secretions in the body *except* Blood, such as saliva, sweat, tears, spinal fluids, and mucus. Fluids are responsible for moistening the skin and muscles, as well as encasing and protecting organ structures. Just like Blood, Fluids can be Deficient or Excess, and they provide excellent clues about overall health.

Hair

Hair doesn't just serve a cosmetic function. It's also a good general indicator of how much Blood and Fluids are circulating through the body. By checking the condition, color, and luster of a patient's hair, I can discover a wealth of things about his or her Lungs, Kidneys, Gall Bladder, and Liver.

If you're suffering a sudden hair loss or premature graying, take heed: they can be warning signs of a condition you may not even be aware of:

- **Premature balding:** Blood Deficiency or natural decline of Qi
- **Bald spot on the crown of your head:** Heat in Liver/Gall Bladder channel
- **Dry, dull hair:** Weak Lungs and Colon, Deficient Blood and Fluids

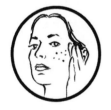

Skin

The color of skin is another indictor of how your body is doing. In fact, all five primary colors can appear on your skin in various degrees: Red, green, yellow, white, and dark blue; each has a direct relationship to various conditions within the body (see page 135). When found in certain areas these colors also give clues to the health of your five power centers. One of the best places to see this is in *skin tones* of the face:

- **Pink skin:** Normal
- **Pale white skin tone:** Energy Deficiency
- **Red skin on the face:** Excessive Heat

- **Yellow skin around the eyes:** Spleen imbalance and Dampness
- **Blue-black skin and circles under the eyes:** Kidney Deficiency

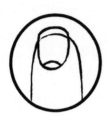

Nails

Nail and nail beds provide further clues. A healthy nail color is a soft shade of pink, but if your nails are showing other telltale signs, I can add it to the emerging physical picture:

- **Light pink nail beds:** Normal
- **Dry, brittle nails:** Liver Deficiency
- **Pale nail beds:** Energy Deficiency
- **Purple and bulging nails:** Heart imbalance

Each is an indication that certain power centers need toning and strengthening. To get even more information, let's move on to the mouth and face.

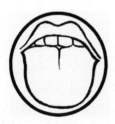

Tongue

The area in and around the mouth is positively loaded with signs of the body's internal condition. By checking the coating, color, and shape of the tongue, we can gather numerous clues necessary for making a comprehensive diagnosis.

The very tip of your tongue tells us how your Heart and Lungs are doing (see figure 8-4). The left and right side of the tongue reveal the health of your Liver and Gall Bladder, while the middle indicates the

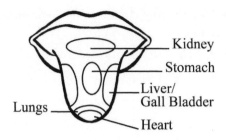

Figure 8-4. Organ Map of the Tongue

Spleen and Stomach conditions. If we look at the very back of the tongue we can see how your Kidneys are functioning.

The symptoms can be many, but here are a few I see in a typical day:

- **Smooth, pink tongue:** Normal
- **Pale, thin tongue with tooth imprints on the side:** General Deficiency
- **Red tongue:** Excessive Heat
- **Purplish, moist tongue:** Cold and Stagnant Blood
- **Swollen tongue:** Internal Dampness, Deficiency
- **Cracked tongue:** Deficiency, weak Heart function
- **Yellow-coated tongue:** Excessive Heat

Lips

The condition of the lips provides an excellent in- 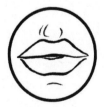 sight into the digestive system, and shows me the amount of energy and fluids available to them.

- **Slightly pink lips:** Normal
- **Cracked lips:** Spleen or Stomach Deficiency

- **Pale lips:** General Deficiency, Lung Deficiency
- **Bright red lips**: Excessive Digestive Heat

Many combinations of symptoms are possible, so we'll need to dig deeper to get a full picture of a patient's health.

Second Examination: Listening and Smelling

In the second phase of the exam I use my ears and nose. By *listening* to your breathing and *smelling* your breath I get a comprehensive snapshot of the Lungs and overall respiratory system. At the same time, my senses are giving me clues to other aspects of your internal and external condition.

Listening

When I hear patients speaking in a loud voice or very rapidly, it usually reveals an excessive amount of Qi. If their voice is halting and whispery soft, there may not be enough Qi to go around. The same clues can be applied to breathing issues. Coughing and secreting a lot of mucus means there is Dampness somewhere in their system. If I hear a parched cough, with an absence of sputum, that's a sure sign of internal Dryness.

Smelling

In modern life we try so hard *not* to give off any smells and yet that is our natural state. Notice the way dogs approach one another and sniff. This is an important way to determine their position in the pack—strong or weak, male or female, the nose says it all. Well, it's not so different than what I do every day. A good sniff can teach me a lot about what issues might be causing a patient's symptoms. Foul, rotten, putrid body or mouth odor indicates a problem with Heat, most likely in the Stomach area. A complete absence of odor usually indicates a Cold condition.

Of course there are a lot of possibilities in between, but by using scent, a fuller story is becoming clear.

Once I've looked and heard and smelled, it's time to ask you, the patient, for your perspective.

Third Examination: Asking

With medical costs so high, most Western doctors don't have time to talk to their patients. As a traditional Chinese doctor, I have to know everything I can about your health and lifestyle habits before I can properly treat a condition. First, I'll ask for a full medical history. If you're working with another doctor, Western or otherwise, it's important that all of us work as a team. I fully believe that every physician—regardless of medical tradition—must join forces in the patient's best interest. I always ask to see the results of any medical tests, in case we need to coordinate with another doctor.

Finally, I'll ask some very specific questions. Some may seem personal, but again, a Chinese doctor can heal only when he or she has the complete picture.

Where Is Your Pain?

Most of my patients come to me because they're feeling some type of discomfort or pain. Where that pain is located often gives me specific information about which power centers are affected. A *pain in the chest*, for example, could mean an imbalance in the Heart, Liver, or Lungs. Pain in the *lower back* often indicates an imbalance of the Kidneys or Bladder.

The *type* of pain is also important. A sharp, stabbing pain can be caused by Stagnation of Blood, while a dull throbbing pain is a sign of a Deficiency somewhere. Also, I want to know how long the pain has been present. Fresh pains, such as muscle strains or tears, often indicate an exterior condition. Long-term chronic pain usually points to a deeper, emotional source.

Do You Sweat?

How many times have you heard, "Never let 'em see you sweat?" In modern society it's considered impolite to let any body odor sneak out. From a young age we're taught to heap on the deodorant and close up those pores. Yes, an odor-free environment has its place, but it's good to remember that sweat is the body's way of releasing toxins.

Perspiration is connected to the health of the Heart, so if you are constantly sweating without exerting yourself physically, it's a good sign that you're experiencing a Deficient condition. On the other hand, if you don't perspire at all, a Cold condition is the probable cause. Night sweats in particular suggest a Deficient condition, whereas excessive sweating during the day can mean you have a Heart or Lung imbalance.

How Is Your Appetite and Thirst?

Asking this question often results in a wealth of valuable health information. Since your ability to process water is ruled by the Kidneys, and your appetite and digestion are controlled by the Stomach and Spleen, eating and drinking habits are an easy way to keep tabs on these two power centers. As you may remember from earlier chapters, a lack of thirst is the sign of a Cold condition, whereas too much thirst is a sign of Heat. An overly abundant appetite also points to Heat, and if nothing on the menu looks good there's probably a Deficiency somewhere.

How Are Your Urine and Stool?

Western medicine puts a lot of emphasis on examining urine and stools for clues to disease, and so does a Chinese physician. The methods vary, though. Instead of chemically analyzing a sample, I rely on color and consistency to assess the state of my patients' overall energy. Pale urine and stools generally indicate a Deficient and Cold condition. Dark yellow and reddish urine suggests Heat and infection.

A normal stool should be firm, so if your stool is dry and hard and you feel constipated, it means there is too much Heat and Deficient Fluid in the Liver or Intestines. Chronic watery stools or diarrhea suggest a possible Deficiency in the Spleen or Kidneys, or possibly an infection in the Colon.

Do You Sleep at Night?

As you've read in earlier chapters, quality rest is crucial for your power centers to operate smoothly. If a patient is having sleep problems, it suggests this person is unable to translate the Yang energy of the day into the Yin energy of the night (see page 197). Abnormal sleep patterns can often be traced directly to problems with the Heart, Kidneys, or Liver and Gall Bladder.

How Is Your Menstrual Cycle?

For women, the health of their menstrual cycle is a key part of my overall diagnosis. This is why I ask detailed questions about the length and consistency of my female patients' periods. A short cycle that occurs twice a month with excessive deep red Blood indicates too much Heat and/or Blood Stagnation. Late, long-lasting periods suggest evidence of a Cold condition and a possible Deficiency. If you experience inordinate amounts of white, vaginal discharge, I can usually pinpoint a Spleen Deficiency. In all of these cases, the characteristics of the menstrual cycle are telling me what is going on deeper in the body.

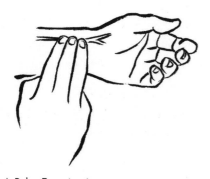

A Pulse Examination

Fourth Examination: Touching

In the last phase of an examination I *feel* the health of your power centers by means of a pulse diagnosis. On the surface, this procedure resembles the motions a Western doctor might use to check your heartbeat. But while a Chinese practitioner does read your pulse, it is in a very different way and for very different results.

When I perform a pulse diagnosis, I'm not just measuring heart rate. It is yet another way to refine all of the information I've gathered from the Looking, Listening, and Asking phases of the examination.

By connecting with my patients' inner rhythms I get an intricate snapshot of each of their five power centers and the strengths and weaknesses of their Qi. I can tell if there is an imbalance, and how

A DOCTOR'S DIAGNOSTIC CHECKLIST

Pain

—Where is it?

—How does it feel?

— Is it sharp or stabbing?

— Is it dull?

— Is it relieved by pressure?

— Is it better with warmth?

— Is it better with cold?

Urine

— Frequency? (Day, night)

— Amount? (Trickle, stream)

— Burning sensation?

— Color (Clear, dark yellow, dark red)

— Urge (Wants to go but can't)

Sweat

—How much?

—Daytime?

—Nighttime?

Stool

—Frequency (Day, night)

—Consistency? (Hard, loose, watery)

—Amount?

—Color (Pale, dark)

—Straining?

Thirst

— Drinks large amounts?

— Drinks nothing at all?

— Craves hot drinks?

— Craves cold drinks?

— Craves sweet drinks?

Sleep

—Difficulty falling asleep?

—Wakes up during night? (Midnight, 3 a.m.)

—Wakes up early morning?

Food

—Eats large amounts?

—Eats nothing at all?

—Craves hot food?

—Craves cold food?

—Craves sweet food?

— Craves spicy food?

Women's Issues

—PMS? (Moody, irritable)

—Breast tenderness?

—Menstruation? (Short or long)

—Period length? (Number of days)

— Irregular?

—Color, clots? (Brown, red, black, deep red)

—Cramps?

superficial or deep it might be. Important information about temperature and blood circulation is noted and added to the bigger picture. This diagnosis is so revealing I can often tell the sex of a baby just by feeling variations in the expectant mother's pulse.

One of my patients put it best: A pulse diagnosis, she said, was like having a full-body MRI without the cost and discomfort.

Reading the Pulse

To begin the exam, I ask patients to rest their left wrist, palm facing up, on a small pillow. I then place my index, middle, and ring fingers on the radial artery of their outer wrist, about an inch from the base of their thumb.

This allows me to read three power centers at one time. On the patient's left hand my index finger feels the Heart energy network; the middle finger, the Liver; and ring finger, the Kidneys. I then switch to the patients' right hand, where I read three more power centers, the Kidneys, the Spleen and Stomach, and the Lungs (see table 8-1).

There are twenty-eight classic pulses a Chinese practitioner must learn. Reading each pulse takes years to perfect. When done properly, a patient will feel the doctor's palpitating three different times

TABLE 8-1. PULSE POSITIONS

My Position	Your Left Hand	Your Right Hand
1. My index finger	Reads your Heart	Reads your Kidney
2. My middle finger	Reads your Liver	Reads your Spleen
3. My ring finger	Reads your Kidney	Reads your Lung

with varying intensities. The goal is to discover which kind of pulse is present and whether a blockage resides close to the surface, or lies deeper within the body.

Basic Pulse Types

Fast or Slow?

In Western medicine, it's considered normal if a pulse hovers at around sixty-eight to seventy-five beats per minute. A traditional Chinese doctor uses a different method. Instead using beats per minute, he or she will synchronize your pulse to your individual breathing patterns. A *normal* pulse rate is four pulses (or beats) per breath at a rate of around eighteen breaths per minute. A *slow* pulse has fewer than four beats per breath and usually indicates a Cold condition. A *fast* pulse usually suggests a Heat pattern.

TEST YOUR PULSE RATE THE CHINESE WAY

Take one long breath in and out. Put three fingers on your radial artery. Take another breath in and out, and count the beats per inhalation and exhalation.

Deep and Floating?

If a pulse is strong under gentle pressure, but grows faint when pushing hard on the artery, this signifies a problem lying somewhere near the surface of the body. We call this a *floating* pulse, and it suggests the patient is experiencing an "attack" from the outside, such as the Five Devils (Heat, Cold, Dry, Damp, and Wind). This can often show up as a flu or virus.

If the pulse feels *deep* and strong when I press hard, I know the problem is more internal in nature and can be due to anything from an infection to a Blood disorder.

LIFE AND DEATH ACCURACY

My great-grandfather, Ding Gangren, was famous throughout China for his razor-sharp pulse diagnosis. His skill was so great he could actually pinpoint the exact date and time when a sick or elderly patient would die.

Empty or Full?

To get a better idea of how much energy my patients have available, I try to determine if their pulse feels weak, or *empty*, or whether it is *full* and pounds like a drum. Empty signifies a Deficiency, whereas a full pulse indicates an Excessive pattern of energy.

Slippery, Choppy, Wiry, or Tight?

Sometimes a person shows a *slippery* pulse. This type of pulse feels smooth, and slips or slithers under my fingers. This is expected in pregnant women because they are carrying extra fluids and Blood to feed the fetus. In others, this indicates Dampness and mucus in the system.

A *choppy* pulse is uneven and rough and tells me there's a Blood or Qi Deficiency, or possibly some Stagnation or blockages are also possible.

A *wiry* pulse feels taut, like a guitar string, and indicates an imbalance within the Liver and Gall Bladder. A *tight* pulse is similar to a wiry pulse, but has more vibration and suggests an Excessive condition.

These are just some of the many possible pulse types and combinations I take under consideration. Placed alongside other phases of a consultation, I can tell which of the five power centers need strengthening, as well as which emotions are most prevalent and how long they've been affecting the person's system. From there I can prescribe the right treatment and begin the road to recovery.

Diagnosis and Treatment

Now that I've narrowed down the root cause of the problem, and I can explain exactly what is happening inside the body, it's my turn to answer my *patients'* questions. Naturally, most want to know why they got sick and what they can do to fix it, or prevent it from happening again. A good doctor should be able to put their mind at ease. I begin with explaining which of their organs are affected and why, and whether their condition is due to weather or if it lies deeper within their energy channels and power centers. I'll advise them to warm or cool their body, to nourish and strengthen power centers, or calm excessive stress. I'll remind them of their emotional history, and how these burdens can affect their organ networks.

For a patient to get the most from any doctor there has to be a meaningful two-way relationship. Once my patients understand what is happening inside their body, fear and anxiety usually fades. That's when we can truly get to work restoring their health.

Whether the pain is due to illness or injury, I'll use all the tools I have available to alleviate their discomfort. Acupuncture, herbal formulas, exercises, diet: All will help clear blockages and toxins as well as mend or heal any breaks or tears.

Once the pain is alleviated, I move on to *strengthening* and *nourishing* the body so that it can withstand future shocks to the system. The goal is for my patients to stay healthy and take control of their *own* health. This is why I suggest positive changes in diet, lifestyle, relaxation, and exercise.

My personal experiences with illness have put me in a unique position to understand exactly what my patients are going through. I know what it feels like when the body breaks down. And I have experienced that incredible feeling when energy returns along with a new lease on life. This miraculous transformation is what I wish for all of my patients.

The following case study is a fine example of just such a transformation.

From Diagnosis to Perfect Health: Lily

Lily was only 40 when she sat down in my office, but already she had been hospitalized a dozen times with asthma attacks so severe she had barely escaped death. She couldn't function without her inhaler for more than four hours at a time, and she had been taking steroids and heavy doses of antibiotics for over fifteen years.

It wasn't hard to conclude that Lily's asthma and breathing issues were connected to a weakened Lung condition. But what was the root cause? Although asthma was the primary symptom, we still needed to consider a number of other possibilities.

First I *looked* at Lily's overall appearance and energy. She was tall, attractive, a bit too thin, with several telltale symptoms; in particular, an overall Deficiency:

- **Limp posture:** Deficiency
- **Cold hands:** Surface areas Cold
- **Red, puffy eyes:** Liver Heat
- **Yellow palms and feet:** Blood Stagnation, Deficiency

- **Tongue shows red tip and sides and crack down the middle:** Heart and Liver imbalance, Body Deficiency
- **Tongue quivers:** Deficiency
- **Pale lips:** Deficiency

Then I *listened* to Lily's voice and received more clues:

- **Soft, low voice:** Deficiency
- **Dry cough, phlegm low in the windpipe:** Kidney Deficiency, Liver Heat
- **Shortness of Breath:** Liver, Kidney, Nervous System

When I *asked* Lily how she was feeling, and where the pain was located, she led me right to the trouble spots:

- **Nasal polyps:** Lung imbalance
- **Chronic bacterial sinus infections:** Lung, Liver involvement
- **Low appetite, anorexic when she was young:** Spleen, Stomach Deficiency
- **Blood in the stool:** Heat
- **Night sweat:** Yin (Blood) Deficiency
- **Insomnia:** Liver, Heart imbalance
- **Stabbing migraines between 1:00 and 3:00 a.m.:** Liver Heat

A pattern was emerging, and though Lily presented herself as thoughtful and pleasant, I suspected she was hiding a lot of troubling emotions. It was time to *read* her pulses for a more definitive diagnosis:

- **Pulse rate slow and weak:** Deficiency, Cold
- **Pulse shape wiry:** Heat, Liver stress
- **Pulse flat and deep:** Emotional trauma rooted in adolescence

Although Lily's primary symptoms were based in her Lungs, all five of her power centers had been affected. Clearly she was suffering from a variety of issues:

- **Deficiency:** Cold hands, pale skin, dark circles, poor posture
- **Liver Heat:** Yellow skin, red eyes, migraines, insomnia
- **Lung Deficiency:** Wheezing, shortness of breath
- **Spleen Deficiency:** Anorexia, low appetite
- **Kidney Deficiency:** Blue-black circles, Phlegm
- **Heart Deficiency:** Insomnia

From this I concluded that the root cause of Lily's asthma and weak Lungs stemmed from her Liver and a condition known as *Liver Qi attacking the Lung.* At some point early in life, she had been overwhelmed by trauma and had taken on far more than she could handle. Her pulses let me know that the primary emotions behind this were anger and grief, feelings she had clearly been holding on to since adolescence.

Establishing a Trust

Since I had never met Lily before our consultation, it was important for me to communicate my findings as gently as possible, so that she could begin the healing process. I told her that I knew her body-kingdom had been at war for so long that it had become energy poor. The Liver, her commander, was raging out of control like an angry dictator. As a result, the Lungs, her queen, could no longer support the Heart, her king, leaving the rest of the kingdom withered and weakened.

Lily seemed surprised, but confirmed nearly everything her body had told me. She had indeed suffered a severe emotional shock as a teen, when her mother died unexpectedly. As a result, she was left in charge of the household and raising her younger siblings. Lily admitted that she had been forced to put off her own wants and needs, things like pursuing an education and attending social events. She was often frustrated and angry, but had held it in her whole life.

These revelations confirmed my diagnosis. Lily was holding in her primary emotional event, the shock and trauma of her mother's untimely passing, and it had lodged in her Lungs, causing their collapse. Anger and Heat were allowed to rise in her Liver, causing a domino effect that weakened the rest of her power centers.

Lily's Treatment

We immediately got to work on strengthening Lily's power centers. This began with biweekly acupuncture sessions, followed by daily herbal teas and meditation to balance her Lung, Liver, and Spleen. Each week we would alter the herbal teas according to her progress.

By our cooling her physical and emotional Heat and nourishing her power centers, Lily's body began to respond. She stopped eating raw foods and salads and switched to warmer, smaller, protein-rich meals. She even added meditation sessions to the day, which helped her sleep through the night.

Soon Lily's tongue and skin tone began to change. The paleness disappeared and was replaced by a healthy pink. Her yellow hands and feet took on a normal color and she began to breathe easier. Best of all, for the first time in years her former energy had finally returned and after a few months, Lily not only tossed out her inhaler, she became a professional flamenco dancer, and now dances up to five hours a day.

Chinese Medicine and Chronic Disease

Lily's case is only one example of the traditional Chinese examination and treatment procedure that has been practiced for at least 3,000 years. Chinese practitioners have had remarkable success with emotion-based illnesses, as well as with serious and chronic diseases that have historically been difficult to treat, diseases such as lupus, diabetes, and fibromyalgia.

DIABETES

Thousands of years ago diabetes was referred to as the *thirsting and wasting disease,* and was diagnosed by the number of ants that were attracted to sugar in the patient's urine. Since then, organizations such as the World Health Organization have found acupuncture and herbs to be effective in managing and treating diabetes.

Age-old Chinese diagnostic techniques are specifically designed to find the location of these conditions and the point to the source of the imbalance. Once that has been determined, it's a straight path to strengthening and nourishing the body back to health.

Fortunately, the world is starting to take notice. Currently, the World Health Organization is compiling comprehensive research and data on diseases that lend themselves to successful acupuncture treatment (see table 8-2, World Health Organization). Along with government licensing of practitioners, we are seeing an exciting and long overdue confirmation that these treatments work and work well.

Again, it's important to emphasize that one healing tradition does not supersede all others. Doctors of every kind should welcome the opportunity to work with other practitioners—Eastern or Western—to create a healing process that is best for the patient.

You and Your Doctor

If there's one key to a successful doctor-patient relationship, it has to be communication. Very simply, talk. Ask questions. Get specific answers. If you're afraid or nervous, say so. Don't be afraid to talk to yourself. Before visiting the doctor, check in with your body. How do you feel? Then tune in after the examination. Are you feeling better? Are you comfortable with your practitioner? Do you trust him or her?

We have a saying in my family that has been handed down from one generation of physicians to the next: "When a person heals, the doctor can only take 30 percent of the credit. The patient is responsible for the other 70 percent." In other words, my role as a doctor is to provide the spark, that extra energy and knowledge that will help a patient begin his or her healing journey. From there it's up to the person to take our relationship of trust and hope and continue down the path toward total health.

DR. TING'S HEALTH ESSENTIALS

TOOLS OF THE TRADE
- Acupuncture
- Herbs
- Moxibustion
- Tui Na

Four Examinations: The four principle stages of a Chinese doctor's examination process.

1. Looking
- Eyes
- Hair
- Skin
- Nails
- Tongue
- Lips

2. Listening and Smelling
- Loud or soft voice
- Foul, rotten odor or odorlessness

3. Asking
- Pain
- Appetite
- Urine
- Stool
- Sleep
- Menstrual cycle

4. Touching: A Chinese doctor distinguishes among twenty-eight different pulse types.

TABLE 8-2. WORLD HEALTH ORGANIZATION APPROVES CHINESE MEDICINE

In controlled clinical trials, the World Health Organization (WHO) has confirmed that acupuncture therapy has proven to be an effective treatment for the following diseases:

Infections
Colds and flu
Bronchitis
Hepatitis

Internal
Poor eyesight
Hypoglycemia
Dizziness
Sinus infection
Herpes
High blood pressure
Sore throat
Ulcers
Hay fever
Hemorrhoids

Dermatological
Asthma
Acne
Eczema

Genito-urinary and Reproductive
Infertility
Impotence
Neuralgia
Premenstrual syndrome (PMS)
Pelvic inflammatory disease
Vaginitis
Irregular period or cramps
Back pain
Morning sickness

Musculo-skeletal Neurological
Arthritis
Sciatica
Frozen shoulder
Tennis elbow
Tendonitis
Bursitis
Stiff neck
Bell's palsy
Trigeminal neuralgia
Stroke
Cerebral palsy
Polio
Sprains

Mental-Emotional
Depression
Anxiety
Headache
Stress
Insomnia

Eyes-Ears-Nose-Throat
Deafness
Ringing in the ear
Ménière's disease
Earaches

9
Following Nature's Phases
The Cycles of Life

Just as the earth travels through time and space, our human body makes its own natural journey through life. Jing is the vital essence we are born with. As we grow, our Jing matures, allowing us to become a healthy adult. Later in life, however, our Jing declines and becomes a precious resource we need to preserve.

During each phase of life, Jing allows our body to go through natural cycles of growth, development, and change. In Chinese medicine we tend to divide this journey into four separate phases—Infancy through Childhood, Puberty through Adolescence, Young Adult through Middle Age, and Middle Age through Senior Years. Each phase has its own specific period of growth and transformation, and each can be honored by maintaining a healthy lifestyle.

Synchronizing your lifestyle to your current phase of life has a positive effect on your health and opens the road to true longevity.

The Four Phases of Life
Phase One: Infancy Through Childhood
INFANCY

An infant's tiny body is in a tremendous state of *growth* and *flux*. Babies eat vast quantities of food in proportion to their body size, creating lots of Qi and Blood, both vital to their development. Their organs and meridians are also growing at an extraordinary rate, making this a delicate time for every infant's immune system.

Because they haven't yet had a chance to build the strength and stamina they'll have when they're older, infants are more susceptible to attack by the Five Temperature Devils—Heat, Cold, Dry, Damp, and Wind. These are the greatest threats to a young and relatively underdeveloped Wei Qi, a good reason to keep them at bay.

YOUR BABY'S EATING HABITS

As any new mother will no doubt agree, an infants' digestion can be a most sensitive process. At this early phase in life, babies' digestive organs have yet to mature. Their Triple Heater is touchy and sensitive, and their Stomach, Spleen, and Kidneys aren't strong enough to process certain foods.

Colic is a stubborn, painful, and often exasperating intestinal condition created by improper development of the colon and intestines. To ease your baby's pain, massage his or her back by gently pinching the bottom of the spine, then slowly moving up the back to the neck along the Governing Vessel (see figure 9-1).

Babies also produce a lot of mucus and Phlegm, further blocking proper digestion. This is why they prefer to eat small amounts frequently throughout the day.

After your baby is weaned from breast milk, I suggest a mixture of easily digestible proteins—meat broths, for instance—along with

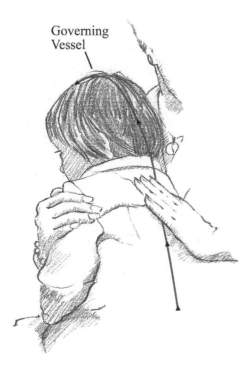

Governing
Vessel

Figure 9-1. Rub along the
Governing Vessel to alleviate
colic and strengthen Qi.

small amounts of well-cooked and pureed fruits and vegetables. I generally recommend that infants do eat some animal protein rather than follow a strictly vegetarian diet for the first few years of their development and growth.

Once again, limit cold foods and drinks. When a child's system has to warm these substances, it forces their power centers to work that much harder.

YOUR BABY'S IMMUNE SYSTEM

As your baby grows, threats to his or her immune system usually show up in external symptoms such as a cold or bronchial infections. These conditions come on quickly and intensely, but can resolve themselves in a relative hurry.

Children are highly susceptible to temperature extremes, so it is vital to keep your baby's power centers warm and dry during the cold months, and cool and protected from heat during the summer months.

If possible, provide your baby with a modified form of my internal organ exercises each morning to strengthen his or her developing immune system (see chapter 3).

Gently rubbing the fingers and toes for example, stimulates all twelve meridian channels. Another important area involves the Governing and Conception Vessels that run up and down the front and back of the body. Massaging these channels also helps stimulate the Lungs, Stomach, and Kidneys.

YOUR BABY'S NERVOUS SYSTEM

Just like adults, babies need to have a reasonable balance between periods of activity (Yang) and rest (Yin). Bombarding a young child with excessive noise, conversation, and electronic stimulation, such as television and videos, only upsets that balance. It can disturb the Shen, leading to memory and attentiveness issues later in life.

Finally, there is nothing better for your baby's health than taking him or her for a stroll in the fresh air. Spending at least thirty minutes each day taking in the five elements will strengthen your baby's power centers and meridian channels. It's fun, and this way the whole family benefits as well.

CHILDHOOD

As the cute tuft of fuzz on your baby's scalp becomes a full head of hair, your child begins to leave the infant stage behind.

The Jing essence regulates this stage of growth. Baby teeth drop out; muscles lengthen, strengthen, and become more flexible. Your child's energy increases dramatically by the day, and those long, peaceful afternoon naps soon become a distant memory.

This is the time when children's Jing starts to amplify and grow, building a firm foundation for a strong body.

Some children, however, have difficulty developing at the rate that they should. It shows up in delayed teething or hair growth, possible stunted physical development. Since Jing resides in the Kidneys, these childhood imbalances are usually a sign of Kidney Deficiency. Often symptoms such as frequent bedwetting are another sign of a Kidney Deficient child.

When I see a young patient with these problems, my job is to strengthen the Kidney through acupressure and herbs. Depending on the age of the child, I guide my patient through a typical diagnosis procedure, including the four steps of Looking, Hearing, Touching, and Asking (see pages 238–253). Since I generally do not use acupuncture on children under the age of ten, I'll create an appropriate prescription, using a combination of Chinese patent pills, herbs, or liquid extracts. Tui Na (Chinese massage) has also lead to excellent results in children of all ages.

BONE SOUP FOR GROWTH AND DEVELOPMENT

YIELD: 3 CUPS

INGREDIENTS:
1/4 POUND BEEF (IF DESIRED)
1 ONION OR 1 BUNCH SCALLIONS, CHOPPED
4 CUPS WATER
1 POUND SLICED BEEF BONES WITH MARROW
1 SLICE GINGER, CHOPPED
ASSORTED CHOPPED VEGETABLES OF CHOICE (CARROTS, CABBAGE, POTATO, TOMATO)

In a 4- to 5-quart pot, sauté the beef, if using, and onion. Add the water, ginger, and bones. Bring to boil. Cover and simmer over low heat for 1 1/2 hours.

Add the vegetables to the pot and cook for an additional 3 minutes. When done, skim the fat, remove the bones, and scoop out the marrow (eat or add to the broth). Serve hot.

YOUR CHILD'S EATING HABITS

We've seen it everywhere: on TV, in magazines—without proper food and nutrients, kids cannot concentrate. From a Chinese perspective the reasons are clear: The Spleen and Stomach are the power centers that fuel concentration, by transforming and sending Blood and Qi to the brain.

These organs aren't just responsible for digestion of food, but of *ideas* and *information.* Feeding children the right foods and strengthening their digestion actually stimulates their ability to learn and process new ideas.

It's a simple principle—when the power centers don't have the fuel to do their job, the body becomes sluggish causing concentration and memory to suffer. If children are making mistakes and doing poorly in school, their emotions will suffer, which can lead to lack of confidence and self-esteem.

If children are experiencing symptoms such as chronic stomach pain, weight gain, headaches, and nausea, or if they have trouble concentrating on schoolwork, it's a possible sign that digestive organs need a boost.

Luckily, there is a lot we can do to help children overcome these difficulties. Since the digestive organs are at their peak during morning and midday hours, it is doubly important that children eat a varied, nutritious breakfast and midmorning snack. A good place to

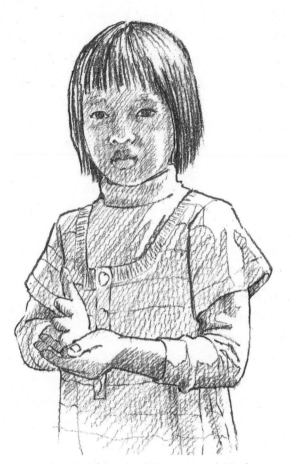

Organ massage can be a helpful tool in helping your child's focus and concentration.

start is with a small serving of protein (egg or cheese), along with some cereal or fruit.

Studies have shown that students who eat breakfast before school do better on exams. In New York and other cities, dramatic improvements have been achieved using groundbreaking pilot programs that feature free breakfast in the classroom.

Hot lunches at noon are also an excellent choice. And when children come home from school, I recommend a healthy snack. They're growing fast, and a bit of energy from a glass of milk can be beneficial before their evening meal. This is also the perfect time to surprise them with that small sugary treat you've been saving all day. At dinnertime keep the meal light, to give their digestive organs the break they need at the end of an energy-filled day.

If digestive symptoms continue to persist, a Chinese doctor can diagnose and prescribe any number of herbal medications, such as Gui Pi Wan (Wake the Spleen Pills), to get those organs working properly.

THE ROOTS OF CHILDHOOD ILLNESS

Every young patient is unique, but in the majority of children I see, Deficiencies in one or more of the power centers are the primary cause: Immune system disorders such as allergies and asthma are nearly always due to a Deficiency in the organ networks.

I begin by carefully assessing your child's health. This means determining his or her unique body patterns and looking for the root cause of the condition. From there I can use various treatments to strengthen the depleted areas.

- **The Kidneys** are in charge of the body's energy supply, while also ruling the health of hair, bones, hearing, and brain activity. So when there isn't enough energy going to this organ, it shows up as hyperactivity and an inability to concentrate.
- **The Heart** houses vital Shen and memory. If this organ becomes imbalanced, it not only affects the child's capacity to recall information but also his or her ability to remain calm.
- **The Liver** reacts strongly to a Deficiency, becoming Hot and Dry and forcing Blood and Qi to circulate at an erratic pace.

This often makes Excessive children react with high levels of anger and frustration, while Deficient children turn inward, becoming more shy and depressed. The extra Heat also leaves them open to bacteria and viruses. This is why cooling and strengthening foods and herbs are often beneficial to a child with this condition.

• **The Spleen** processes nutrition from food, then uses it to fortify Blood and Fluids. To be able to focus, children need this fortification. If yours are picky eaters, it can be evidence of a Spleen Deficiency.

• **The Lungs are** in charge of our protective Wei Qi and regulate the opening and closing of the pores of the skin. If they are weak, children can become prone to skin rashes and eczema as well as chronic respiratory illnesses.

If your children have been showing any of these signs and symptoms for more than a few months, consider taking them to a practitioner to have them evaluated. You could start off with a few gentle herbal formulas and some simple diet tips, and go from there. Chinese medicine has had excellent results in treating everything from Attention deficit disorder (ADD), childhood asthma, and other immune-related diseases.

ATTENTION DEFICIT DISORDER

ADD and attention-deficit/hyperactivity disorder (ADHD) can encompass a broad range of symptoms including irritability, impulsiveness, unruly behavior, and of course, a lack of concentration. Chinese medicine considers ADD as a *Deficiency* (attention *Deficit* disorder) in one or more of the five power centers. Although Western drugs such as Ritalin have proven to be quite effective, long-term use can sometimes lead to side effects. Traditional

Chinese medicine has proven to be an gentler, effective complementary treatment in many cases.

MAINTAINING A PEACEFUL HOME FOR YOUR CHILD

It seems obvious, but patients are sometimes surprised to hear that the psychological and emotional environment of their home can affect their child's health. It's a simple example of cause and effect. Remember, your power centers are quite reactive, not only to internal and external factors, but also to the emotional ebbs and flows of life.

Here are some general recommendations that are easy to remember, and that the whole family will benefit from.

- **Give the gift of touch.** Patting or massaging children—along the spine and Governing Vessel—is one way to access every organ system in their body.
- **Avoid excessive sweets.** Sugar is overly warming and creates extra Heat, which can fuel anger and frustration.
- **Eat strengthening, protein-rich foods.** Children with a Deficiency need the right fuel in the tank. And be sure to have them drink at least four glasses of water per day.
- **Limit TV and video games.** Kids concentrate at school, draining Blood and Qi and putting a strain on their power centers, specifically the Spleen and Stomach network. Add homework and it's easy to see how their mental focus can be challenged. This is why excessive amounts of television or computer games should not be piled upon a long school day. Hyperstimulation and concentration overworks a young mind and leads to sluggish digestion. No child likes to hear this, but placing a reasonable limit on TV and computer

privileges is an effective way to keep children's power centers running smoothly.

- **Remain active.** Adults call it exercise, but children should call it fun. It might be running, playing ball, or team sports, but whatever the activity, it should be something your children enjoy. Even a half hour of vigorous activity is beneficial for proper development and maintenance of Blood, Qi, and critical organs.

- **Slow Down.** If you find yourself constantly rushing through the day, it's time to cut back and pay heed to your Liver. Try some of the exercises and meditation tips mentioned in earlier chapters. Calm parents lead to a calm family.

- **Create a balanced, peaceful environment.** This is easier said than done. But if you can, target at least one day a week where activities are less hectic and you engage in some family activities. Also, arrange your children's study and sleeping space according to the principles of Feng Shui.

Phase Two: Puberty Through Adolescence

As children reach puberty, their body is still in a vigorous growth phase, but now the emphasis is on *building strength* and *stamina*. Emotionally, this is a difficult period, as adolescents are trying to figure out how they fit into a larger world. It's also a period of great change within the body-kingdom.

During puberty, teens' organs and organ systems are preparing for sexual activity. Breasts grow larger, genital organs mature, voices change, and sexual desire intensifies. Teenagers are churning out hormones eight times faster than adults do. Power centers are now working overtime, making this the most intense period of growth in all of life's four phases.

The two organs most affected by this activity are the Liver and Kidneys. The Kidneys and their Jing Qi oversee growth and development and are responsible for producing reproductive hormones. The Liver is charged with circulating those hormones throughout the body.

Teens love to try forbidden things, but if poor nutrition or destructive lifestyle habits interrupt the natural flow, the Kidneys will become Deficient or Liver function will be strained. Either way, the result is hormonal fluids that circulate in jumps and starts, leading to erratic behavior.

TEEN AILMENTS: ACNE AND MIGRAINES

Who doesn't cringe at the memory of an ugly pimple popping up right before that all-important date? In retrospect, it may seem amusing, but at the time it was mortifying. Teen acne can be an embarrassing and isolating problem, leading to a crippling loss of self-esteem.

I know of one American dermatologist who, before effective medicines were available, successfully treated adolescent patients by talking them through the issues they were having at school and home. He found that once they had released some of their anxiety, the acne would disappear.

This confirms what I have seen throughout my practice—that there is usually an emotional component to nearly every health condition, even acne.

Luckily, Chinese medicine has had great success in treating this condition. Setting emotion aside for a moment, the physical causes of acne are typically due to excessive Heat in the body. This Heat can be worsened by stress, frustration, or anxiety, as well as by overconsuming the Heat-inducing sodas and candy that teenagers love. Spicy foods and alcohol are other likely culprits. If we look closely, we can even see that acne breakouts often fall directly on the Stom-

ach or Liver meridian closely following the jaw line right up to the
cheeks (see figure 9-2).

Unlike the Western treatments,
which rely on antibiotic ointments
and pills, Chinese medicine treats
patients according to their unique
energy pattern. This means adjusting acupuncture sessions to target
the root cause of the skin problem.
Herbal formulas, too, must be created for the particular outbreak.

With this treatment, teens usually experience a complete reversal
of symptoms within a few months.
But it doesn't come without some
sacrifice. For the cure to work, they
must cut back on fast foods and follow the guidelines for Neutral and

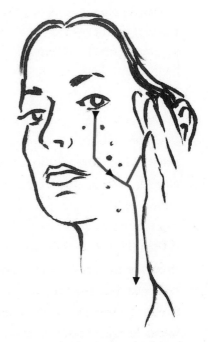

Figure 9-2. Acne Outbreak Along the
Stomach Meridian

Cooling foods, such as cucumber and papaya (see pages 100–101).
Keeping inner Heat in check through diet is vital. Refrain from providing your adolescent sugary and caffeine-based foods, and focus
on protein-rich, strengthening meals. If your teen will try it, regular
yoga or calming meditation definitely helps, too.

TEEN MIGRAINES

Over the last couple of decades, I have seen a sharp increase of adolescent migraines in my practice. Migraines are due to overall Deficiencies or
weakness in the organs, and usually have an emotional trigger. In many
cases, the Liver becomes too Hot and Dry, and the excess Heat rises,
causing headaches and pain. In teenage girls, it is often exacerbated

when meals are skipped in effort to watch weight. In addition to acupuncture and herbal therapies, there are many simple home remedies to maintain and prevent such symptoms: a daily massage of the Liver and Gall Bladder meridians, a color meditation for the Liver, and EFT, to name a few.

TEEN EMOTIONS

Most parents are all too familiar with the stony stares, the sullen glances, and all those unprovoked fits of teen rage. When your happy-go-lucky child suddenly transforms into a teeth-gnashing vampire overnight, it might be time to smooth out the energy flow.

Traditional Chinese medicine emphasizes that feelings and emotions are held and controlled by the power centers. When young teenagers go through puberty, they don't always know how to confront the changes occurring in their body. With the Liver giving off bursts of anger and frustration, and the Kidneys sending spikes of irrational fear, it's no wonder strong emotions are quick to surface.

If this sounds like your teen, a Chinese practitioner can help with acupuncture and a custom herbal formula. or perhaps prescribe Xiao Yao Wan (Free and Easy Wanderer), an effective patent formula to soothe symptoms of anger and depression. This also helps the Liver to function at an even pace.

Keep in mind, though, this age may be challenging, and it's important and healthy for teens to express and release their feelings. Left bottled up, these emotions can cause energy blockages in the body and only worsen behavior. Talk to your teen about how he or she is feeling, even if it means an angry outburst. Allowing adolescents an outlet helps them manage their health.

TEEN DIET

Around the age of fourteen, the digestive system has fully matured. Armed with an active body that is still growing and developing, the average teen requires ample food to keep going. But that doesn't necessarily mean ordering everything at the food court.

In spite of their bottomless appetite, it's important for teens to match portion size with their actual needs. An 80-pound girl shouldn't dig into the same five-course dinner as a 160-pound wrestler. Because adolescents' digestive organs are still getting used to working at an adult pace, excess fast food and oily meals can build up too much Stomach Fire and Heat in their body, leading to migraines, an explosive temper, and weight gain.

Teenagers also tend to skip meals, which can be just as chaotic for the body. Eating habits should be consistent for the Qi to flow rhythmically and efficiently. By eating in stops and starts, they are short-circuiting the process necessary to create Qi and Blood.

To steer kids to the right food choices, adults have to set an example. If children grow up watching parents eat a healthy meal, it's more likely that at least some of the time they'll ignore those unhealthy temptations.

This makes the teen years a perfect opportunity to learn how to cook. I know this from personal experience. Before my father died and my mother took over the family medical practice, I wasn't included in day-to-day meal preparation. Then all at once the family's cooking duties fell on my shoulders. To my surprise I liked it, and I continue to rely on those cooking skills today. By teaching your children to prepare a meal, you are helping them to become self-sufficient. My Easy Beef Stew recipe is a great place to start (see page 278). They will have the ability to create their own Qi, a gift that will last the rest of their life.

INCREASE YOUR ENERGY INCOME:
ESTHER'S EASY BEEF STEW

YIELD: 3 CUPS

INGREDIENTS:
1 POUND BEEF, CUT INTO CHUNKS*
1 LARGE ONION, CHOPPED
3 CARROTS, CHOPPED
4 CUPS WATER
PINCH OF SALT
SUGAR
KETCHUP

Bring the beef, onion, carrots, and water to a boil, then simmer uncovered until the beef and vegetables are tender, about 40 minutes. Add a pinch of salt, sugar, and ketchup to taste. The broth should be a thick paste. Serve the vegetables, beef, and broth over pasta or rice.

*Note: If you prefer, substitute a 14-ounce can of black beans or kidney beans.

TEENS AND EXERCISE

Staying healthy and fit is crucial at any time, especially during the teen years. Throughout childhood and adolescence, young people are building a foundation for adulthood. Growing muscles and tendons are controlled by the Spleen and Liver.

If overused, these important connective tissues can put a heavy strain on a teen's power centers, leading to negative consequences later in life.

That's why it's so important that the intensity of a teen's physical training matches the energy (Blood and Qi) that he or she has available.

I'm a big believer in athletic coaching, and most children have a positive experience with their coaches. Training and team sports are

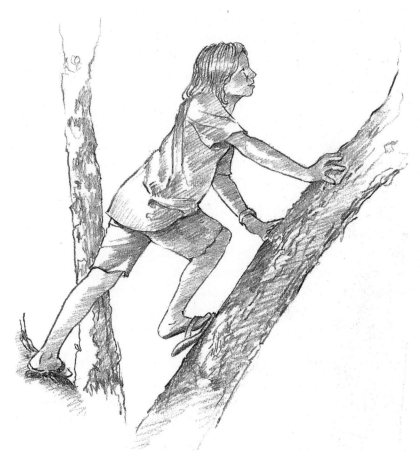

Keep your teen's exercise positive and fun.

great ways to keep young people active. However, parents need to be aware of their teen's endurance and strength-building regimens and ensure that they are always done under proper supervision.

With teenagers playing at ever more competitive levels, some are training more intensely and at younger ages. Again, I can't stress enough the value of moderation.

Usually there are clear signs when excessive training regimens have pushed young people past their limits. If normally active teens show signs of exhaustion, their skin and nails appear pale, and they're overly susceptible to cold or flu. These are generally indications of an underlying energy Deficiency.

Such symptoms are a reliable gauge that your teen should limit his or her exercise and give his or her body a chance to recover.

TEENS AND SEX

The beginning of the reproductive cycle is an important time of life. For girls it's said that their Jing Qi matures when menstruation begins, although this is not the whole story. A girl may technically be able to conceive in her teens, but her reproductive cycle is not fully mature until at least the age of twenty-one.

Males are a bit different. According to the *Nei Jing*, boys' reproductive cycles mature at age sixteen, when they are already prepared to become sexually active. This cycle peaks and matures at the age of twenty-four.

Chinese medicine emphasizes a strong link between early sex and health problems. Sexual activity is ruled by the Kidneys. Having frequent sex throws a young body off balance, depleting energy and forcing the organs to work overtime to compensate for this loss. Remember that the Kidneys also rule brain growth and development. Any excess strain on these organs affects brain power and causes memory loss.

From a Chinese medical standpoint, I believe that abstaining from sex until after high school is a good idea. Although it might seem unrealistic in light of today's sexually active teens, there's a sound reason. Since their Kidney Jing Qi doesn't peak until their early twenties, adolescents' power centers aren't equipped to handle the physical and emotional stress that a sexual relationship imposes on them.

Western science is starting to confirm this view. Ohio State University's recent studies support what Chinese medicine has known all along: that kids who wait until after they are seventeen are much less likely to have academic difficulties, commit crimes, smoke, or suffer from emotional problems.

We need to encourage and support this physical and behavioral transition in adolescents in whatever way we can. This means giving them the tools to build a strong mental, physical, and spiritual foundation.

Pay attention to what your teen is watching on television and visiting on the Internet, and stay abreast of his or her social and romantic relationships.

Finally, talk to your adolescent about sex. If you feel he or she needs a neutral environment to share such issues, find a support group in your area (see the resources section).

TEEN ABSTINENCE

According to a recent study by Ohio State University, teens who become sexually active earlier than their peers (ages 13 through 17) are much more likely to steal, destroy property, and participate in drug culture than do those who wait.

Phase Three: Young Adult Through Middle Age

As you age from a young adult to your middle years, you come to the most powerful phase in life's journey. This is the age when women are their most fertile and men their most potent.

Phase three is a highly active period. By now you probably have a career and family of your own, and you need the stamina to maintain

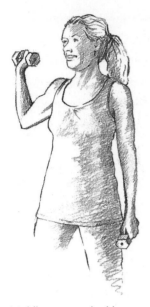

Middle age is a highly active period.

them. Your body is supple and strong; your entire energy system is operating at its peak.

With all this added responsibility our energy reserves need to be carefully managed.

It's probably not a surprise that adult men and women deal with their health issues differently. I see it in my practice all the time. Men tend to bottle up any pressure they feel from their heavy responsibility. They hide their health issues and are hesitant to come in for treatment. Adult women, on the other hand, often feel they can't afford the time to slow down and make the changes necessary to ensure proper health.

If we look at each sex individually, we can see the reasons for these differences. According to ancient theory, Kidney Qi matures and develops using a slightly different growth cycle in men and women. Whereas a woman's Qi surges and wanes on a seven-year cycle, a man's body works on an eight-year cycle (see table 9-1).

Of course, modern medical and nutritional advances have made it possible to increase well beyond these ancient guidelines. I reference them here to bring home an important point: It's common knowledge that most women reach menopause in their mid- to late forties; but men, too, go through their own form of menopause when their Kidney Jing declines.

Let's compare the sexes.

Adult Men: A Chinese Perspective

Ask any woman and she'll probably agree that most men tend to disregard the changes in their body, even when they are being sent a

TABLE 9-1. THE RISE AND FALL OF KIDNEY QI
ACCORDING TO THE *NEI JING*

MEN 8–Year Cycle	WOMEN 7–Year Cycle
0–8 Qi is growing, hair, permanent teeth arrive.	0–7 Qi is growing, hair, permanent teeth arrive.
8–16 Blood and Qi grow and prosper.	7–14 Blood and Qi grow and prosper.
16–24 Puberty begins and matures.	14–21 Puberty and menstruation begin.
24–32 Kidney Qi peaks and matures, sexual activity begins, peak physical condition.	21–28 Kidney Qi peaks and matures; most fertile years, peak physical condition.
32–40 Blood and Qi begin natural decline.	28–35 Tendons, bones strong, body developed.
40–48 Hair thins and turns gray, skin wrinkles.	35–42 Blood and Qi begin natural decline.
48–56 Muscles, tendons weaken.	42–49 Menstruation ceases, hair thins and turns gray, skin wrinkles.
	49–56 Muscles, tendons weaken, ability to conceive ceases.

clear message. They ignore discomfort and pain, often postponing a checkup. I hear the same reasons all the time: "It's too expensive . . . My family and kids come first . . . If my colleagues think I'm sick, my job could be jeopardized." As a result, they postpone seeing me until the symptoms become too much to bear.

What I would like men to understand is that Chinese medicine doesn't just treat their symptoms, it roots out the reasons for those symptoms. By looking into both the physical and emotional causes of a health problem, I can usually find a number of related issues. In fact, many men come in with one complaint and later discover other problems they hadn't even considered.

Men face ailments ranging from infertility to prostate problems. Chinese medicine has had great success with many of these conditions.

A low sperm count can be the sign of a hot Liver, which can lead to tense muscles. A stomach ulcer can be caused by a weak Spleen, which can result in migraine headaches. It's a fundamental link that often surprises many of my male patients.

Many of these conditions can be illuminated by looking at processes specific to the male body.

ACUPUNCTURE HEALS LOW SPERM COUNT: ANTONIO

Antonio first walked into my office complaining of a back problem that had been bothering him for over a year. He'd been on several painkillers and had spent countless hours in physical therapy. While examining him, I found energy blockages that were centered in his upper back. His symptoms were the result of Heat radiating from the Liver and Gall Bladder channels. I wasn't surprised. Antonio was a man who took his job seriously and had been putting himself under a lot of pressure to perform.

I treated Antonio for some months and eventually freed him from his back pain. He returned a few times for a virus or flu, not knowing his biggest health challenge was still ahead of him.

One day Antonio came to see me, looking despondent. When I asked why, it turned out that he and his wife had just learned they couldn't conceive. His sperm count was extremely low, and the doctor told him to consider other options.

We began treatment by focusing on strengthening his Kidneys, the power center in charge of sexual reproduction. As I suspected, the root cause of Antonio's low sperm count was exactly the same villain I had diagnosed a few years earlier: excessive Liver Heat. Antonio was producing so much Heat that his sperm literally "burned up" before they could properly form.

We began a regimen of cooling and nourishing herbal teas, and within a week his sperm count had jumped from 1 million to 25 million. After three sessions I got the happy news that his wife had become pregnant. As a side benefit of the herbs, Antonio lost twenty pounds and saw his seasonal colds and allergies disappear. He also felt much calmer and less stressed.

This is a perfect example of how Chinese medicine can make a difference in a relatively short time. It can be just as effective for male problems where surgery is recommended as the first choice.

SURGERY AVOIDED: SCOTT

Recently, Scott came to see me for an enlarged testicle. Naturally, he was upset because his internist had diagnosed a tumor and was recommending surgery to remove it. My diagnosis told me the enlargement wasn't a growth after all. It turned out to be accumulated Heat that had created inflammation and infection. I asked if he was willing to put surgery on hold for a few weeks and let me treat him. After a regimen of anti-inflammatory herbs to eradicate the infection,

Scott recovered completely, all without ever risking the dangers of surgery.

SYMPTOMS OF THE PROSTATE

In newborn males, the prostate is the size of a pea and grows from there. By the time a man reaches his late twenties, it has become the size of an average walnut. Then middle age rolls around, and several common problems can cause the prostate to swell and become painful, among them prostatitis and benign prostatic hyperplasia (BPH).

I'll begin by giving my patient a full pulse examination. If I suspect problems with the prostate, I'm most likely to concentrate on the organ systems and meridians that intersect the prostate and male genitals—in this case the Kidney, Liver, and Governing Vessel. By clearing the residual Heat, toxins, and stagnant Qi, circulation improves, reducing inflammation and eliminating pain and discomfort.

My advice to men is simple: If you know there's something wrong inside your body-kingdom, take care of it. Don't ignore those aches and pains; listen to them. More often than not, they're trying to tell you something you should hear.

Adult Women: A Chinese Perspective

Throughout my career, I've treated women of all sizes, ages, and phases of life.

For most of my female patients, the period between young adult and middle age is often their busiest and most eventful. Their bodies and emotions have experienced everything from childbirth to divorce, and sometimes their health has suffered.

By the time my female patients come to see me, they're often depressed and in pain, and have been suffering for a long time. They're nervous about the diagnosis, and afraid to be classified with a "disease" or a condition for which there is no hope. Time and again, these anxious emotions do more harm to their body than do the physical symptoms they are experiencing.

If only these patients could see what I see—that most gynecological conditions are caused by four basic issues: Blood Stagnation, Blood Deficiency, poor diet, and emotional stress.

Luckily, Chinese medicine has had extensive experience with these symptoms. In fact, one of the most comprehensive textbooks on women's obstetrics and gynecology was published in China in AD 600, predating Western medical texts by at least seventeen hundred years.

When a female patient asks me what a Chinese doctor can do, I always give the same answer. It's not just what *I* can do, but how Chinese medicine can be harnessed to stimulate *her own* healing abilities. Together we need to redirect and fortify the patient's Blood and Qi, then strengthen and balance the power centers and emotions, so that her body can function normally.

A CURE FOR ENDOMETRIOSIS: KANESHA

She arrived in my office suffering from severe endometriosis. Kanesha, 29, had already put herself through the ringer: injections, antibiotics, even surgery. Despite these treatments, Kanesha's pain persisted. She was forced to quit her job in the South and move to Los Angeles so that her mother could help with her medical care.

The diagnosis was devastating. Western doctors had warned her that it would be difficult, if not impossible, for her to conceive, a fate she would have to accept.

After listening to Kanesha's heartbreaking story, my initial goal was to relieve her pain. Since Kanesha was nearing her peak reproductive years, we would also need to rebalance her organs so that she could one day conceive when she felt ready.

My examination revealed a great deal of pent-up frustration, which Kanesha confirmed. The premature loss of her father and her hectic workload as a customer service rep had created a lot of stress. All of this had created a backlog of emotional Heat and constriction in Kanesha's Blood vessels. Overweight and living on a unhealthy diet of hot, greasy foods, she was experiencing gas, cramping, and debilitating digestive and urinary issues.

From a Chinese perspective, endometriosis is a condition caused by Blood Stagnation, involving the Liver, which is in charge of regulating the volume of Blood and Qi. The Kidneys, which are in charge of reproduction and birth, also play a part. When we say the Blood stagnates, this means that its flow is decreased by obstructions or *tension* in the blood vessels.

Kanesha and I began working together to cool her inner Heat and strengthen her Kidneys and Liver. After a few weeks she felt better, but her real progress came after she finally released years of emotional anxiety and pain. Kanesha went from taking ten pills a day to needing none at all. As a side benefit, she lost weight, and returned to work a few months later. Kanesha now owns her own business and is looking forward to finding a partner and starting a family of her own.

LONG-LASTING RELIEF FROM IRREGULAR PERIODS: MARIA

Irregular menstrual cycles are fairly common so it wasn't unusual that Maria's doctors had put her on the pill to ease her symptoms. In her case, however, it wasn't helping. In addition to painful and irregular periods, Maria was suffering side effects: a bloated stomach and bad acne, as well as overwhelming feelings of instability.

Menstruation can be a difficult time for women. During the monthly cycle, excess Blood is filtered by the Liver, pushing it to work at full capacity. Irritability and anger often results, bringing on a build up of gas in the blood vessels, typically leading to cramps and stomach pains.

The Liver has another connection to menstrual periods. Meridians run from the big toe to the upper chest, passing over and through the reproductive organs (see figure 9-3). Since the Liver and Gall Bladder are responsible for strategy and decision making, menstrual periods are a good time to hold off on big decisions until the cycle is over and the Liver is back to normal.

Western medicine prescribes birth control pills as a cure-all for irregular menstruation as well as many other gynecological conditions. Although this may be a necessary course for many women, Chinese medicine approaches contraceptives more cautiously. Chemical birth control has a very strong influence on the energy channels. Over time it can damage the reproductive cycle and stop the natural function and flow of hormones in the uterus. This doesn't just affect fertility and related functions, it can also harm the body's power centers.

Contraceptive chemicals also have a harsh *drying* effect on the Liver. As Maria was already suffering from Liver Heat, the pill, in effect, was adding fuel to the fire. The excess Heat moved upward toward her Lungs, and, because the skin is a sister organ related to the Lungs, the Heat began causing acne eruptions along the Liver channels in her face.

I took Maria off the contraceptives and used herbs to cool her Liver, Kidneys, and Lungs. Her menstrual flow responded, returning to normal, and soon thereafter, her bloating disappeared. In addition,

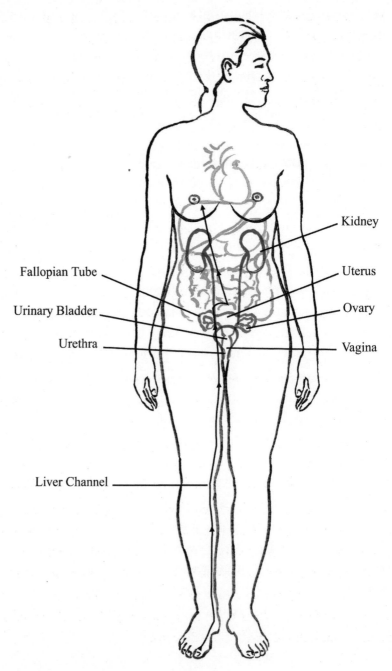

Kidney

Fallopian Tube

Uterus

Urinary Bladder

Ovary

Urethra

Vagina

Liver Channel

Figure 9-3. The Liver meridian passes over the sexual organs.

we eliminated spicy, greasy foods from her diet and switched to smaller, warmer meals. Maria's acne cleared up completely and she felt better within a matter of weeks. The recipe for success wasn't difficult. When the Liver, Kidneys, and Lungs were calm and cool, they were able to rebalance and move back into a regular rhythm and flow.

RELAXATION EASES CONCEPTION: ELAINE

Elaine was near tears. It was our first appointment together, and even before I had started my diagnosis, her distress came spilling out of her: She wanted to have a child, but no matter how hard she tried, her thirty-five year old body refused to cooperate. It wasn't the first time I had heard the statement, "My biological clock is ticking, and I'm running out of time." Elaine was desperate for help.

As it turned out, Elaine's Western doctor had given her a clean bill of health. She *should* have been able to conceive and yet she and her husband had not been able to do so. I was their last ray of hope before starting the difficult and costly process of artificial insemination.

The first thing Elaine wanted to know was, "Why is my body fighting me?"

After a full diagnosis, I was fairly sure I knew the answer. It was right there in her pulse: the perfect example of an Excessive patient. After questioning her further, my initial diagnosis was confirmed. Elaine was a busy, high-powered lawyer who was used to getting things done her way. Her Liver was hot, tense, and tight—typical symptoms of people who stretch themselves beyond their limits.

To create the right conditions for the coupling of egg and sperm, sex should be enjoyed in a calm, stress-free environment. It's only under these circumstances that the primary ingredients of a successful pregnancy, Blood and Qi, can flow freely.

"I know you are determined to have a child," I told her, "but right now it's necessary to focus on yourself. For the next few weeks I want you to treat your body with the same tender care as you would give your own baby. "

Elaine's job was simple. First, she needed to calm down and relax. This would immediately help her Blood, Qi, and reproductive fluids, all of which were experiencing intense Heat. This was the same Heat that was "burning" her husband's sperm before it had a chance to fertilize.

Elaine needed to put aside the worries and pressures of her job, at least for a while, and spend some relaxing time with her spouse.

Taking my suggestions to heart, she and her husband added some relaxation exercises to their day. She also responded well to treatments of acupuncture and cooling herbs, and within just a few weeks they were able to conceive.

PREGNANCY AND HEALTH

Because pregnancy and childbirth particularly affects the strength of the Kidneys, Liver, and Spleen, it is vitally important that women protect and strengthen these power centers before and after childbirth. Stock up on easily digested, protein-rich foods, such as soups and stews, and make time for plenty of rest. Acupuncture, herbs and Tui Na have proven to be very effective treatments before, during, and after pregnancy.

Most of the younger women I treat anticipate the profound changes their body will go through during pregnancy. I always urge that they pay close attention to the telltale signs and nurture their body in a loving way before those changes come. In this way nature will help them make the transition with ease and grace.

Menopause: A Natural Decline of Qi

When I moved to the United States, I was a forty-two-year-old single mother with a hundred dollars in my pocket. I was thrilled to be living in what I call my "earthly heaven," my adopted hometown of Santa Monica, California. But the early pressures to survive were overwhelming. Although my sister Rhoda and my sponsor family did everything they could to help, I still had to learn English and support my young son and myself. Many years of hard work were in store for me before I could build a financial and social foundation that would allow me to start my own practice.

It was a difficult and stressful journey but, five years later, I finally had my own apartment and car. I had even started a makeshift practice in a spare bedroom at home. But in spite of all my good fortune, I was cranky and irritable. I wasn't learning English fast enough and the certification process was taking too long. No matter how hard I tried, I never seemed to get enough sleep. I was either too hot or too cold, and many nights I woke up sweating profusely.

One morning it all became so clear. My son, Peter, looked at me across the breakfast table and asked, "Why is Mommy always upset?" That's when I knew it was time to take a good, hard look at myself.

At the age of forty-seven I was stressed and tired. More important, I wasn't paying attention to where I was at this midpoint in my life cycle. I wasn't listening to my body. I had lost touch with my physical and emotional being.

It wasn't an easy thing to do, but I needed to slow down, simplify my expectations, and give my body the break it desperately needed to move through this "change of life."

For women, menopause is a natural part of the Qi cycle. The ages from forty-eight to fifty-five years of age mark the time when a woman's vital essence, or Jing, transitions from a period of growth to

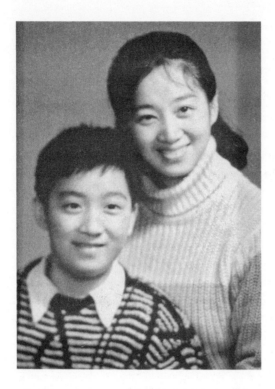

My son, Peter, and I in 1982, right before we came to the United States. I was forty-two and had been practicing Chinese medicine in my native country for twelve years.

a gentle decline. As hormone production wanes and ovulation ceases, women often experience hot flashes, headaches, vaginal dryness, and insomnia. Psychological side effects such as agitation, depression, and memory lapses may also occur. All of this is due to a natural Deficiency in the Kidneys and Liver.

Treatment for menopause or similar Deficiencies should include the remedies covered in this book: Daily internal organ exercises (see chapter 3), visualization and meditation (see chapter 5), as well as a diet featuring neutral and strengthening foods (see chapter 4).

A woman's ultimate success, however, depends on making lifestyle changes that support her health. Alleviating emotional stress is a crucial part of making that come true.

I understand that this is easier said than done. Life has a way of throwing mountains to climb at the very time a person needs to be coasting downhill. All I ask is that you anticipate the potential stress brought on by middle age and take control before your power centers feel the heat.

And if you do find yourself experiencing uncomfortable or painful symptoms, remember that a Chinese practitioner can evaluate these problems and recommend a course of action. Without resorting to strong drugs, Chinese medicine can ease this transitional period with a number of acupuncture and herbal treatments that specifically target the changes that menopause brings.

MARIANNE JAS'S STORY: THE MIDLIFE MAMBO

After eight difficult years it seemed as if I had finally put my health issues behind me, and I felt I could finally move on with my life.

Not so fast.

It began the day I turned forty-eight years old—severe hot flashes that appeared every half hour for 24-hour periods. They went on for weeks and brought with them perspiration, hair loss, disturbed sleep, and insomnia. Once again I found myself confused and distraught. It felt as if my former chronic fatigue symptoms had returned for another round. Even more depressing was that despite all my newfound knowledge of herbs, remedies, and acupressure points, I seemed unable to help myself.

One morning, following yet another endless night with no sleep, I found myself hugging my husband's knees, crying in despair. He rubbed my back, gave me a little smile, and said brightly, "Why don't you go see Esther?"

When I compared notes with friends in the same situation, they warned me to prepare for long, expensive hormone treatments that could last weeks if not months. Not exactly an appealing prospect. Okay, Esther it was.

She sat me down and ran through her by-now familiar examination. Was it bad? Would I be put on a strict diet with multiple herbs? "No big deal, Marianne." She smiled. "You are nearing the beginning of a new cycle. These hot flashes are simply caused by spikes in temperature, a temporary Yin Deficiency brought on by the natural decline of Jing in the Kidneys."

She explained that my spikes in temperature were merely a temporary Yin Deficiency due to the natural decline of Jing in the Kidneys.

In Chinese medicine hormones are considered a part of the Fluids that course through the body. During menopause these Fluids and vital Blood are lacking, leaving fewer hormones to go around. This is why the system needs to be rebalanced.

Esther prescribed cooling and strengthening herbs, and advised me to rest and to eat protein-rich meals to strengthen my Blood and Fluids.

Sure enough, after one week, the hot flashes had subsided. And since that time, no major flare-ups have returned.

Another key component in my "second" recovery was following this daily regimen:

- The herbal formula Lieu Wei Di Huang Wan to nourish the Kidneys
- Daily meditation and EFT
- 6 cups of water with lemon
- 6 small protein meals and snacks, with my main meal at midday
- A cup of warm milk or almond milk with protein powder in the afternoon and at bedtime
- Seven hours' rest a night

Instead of dreading midlife, I feel calm and relaxed and confident—knowing how to take care of myself during this transitional period.

Phase Four: Middle Through Senior Years

As people move into their fifties, the next phase of life begins: the middle through senior years. Their Jing starts to slowly decline and the body begins showing the signs. Hair starts to gray, joints and muscles lose some of their elasticity, and female reproductive organs surrender their ability to conceive.

With less Jing, men and women now have fewer guards to protect their body-kingdom. Their Wei Qi is also diminishing, and they lose a small portion of their ability to fight off disease. This makes it important to *protect* and *preserve* their precious vital essences and keep their immune system strong.

Chinese medicine can certainly counteract some of this loss.

Remember that your energy bank account is made up of two currencies: (1) your Inherited Qi, or Jing; and (2) your Acquired Qi, the energy you receive from food and exercise. By eating a healthy and energy-rich diet, fortifying your Blood with oxygen, and balancing it with appropriate rest, you can actually "top up" your energy reserves and prolong life. I am now seventy-two and still go to dance class four times a week. By following this simple regimen, I feel healthier than I did in my thirties!

Let's see what you can do to make the fourth phase of life as rewarding as the others.

SENIOR DIGESTION AND DIET

As Jing declines, the digestive process has less energy available. Without that power, your Spleen and Stomach are still working hard but with diminished resources. But you can help by making deposits of fresh energy—energy that will power your digestion even as you age.

Many seniors feel bloated and overweight. Others are undernourished and have no appetite at all. These conditions happen because their digestive factory doesn't have enough energy to transform the nutrients from food, an excellent reason to eat the right foods at the right times.

The other advice I give older patients is to modify the *way* they're eating. Many seniors continue shoving their meals down as if they're in a race. In this phase of life it's wise to give the digestive organs a break. Slow down, enjoy each bite, and consider going back to some of the eating habits from infancy.

Again, avoid greasy, spicy, and sugary foods. Eat smaller, warmer meals. Remember, your digestive plant needs less energy to transform a warm meal into Blood and Qi than it does a meal of cold, raw foods. Drink Bone Soup (see page 267) to give your Kidneys and bones a boost, or my Easy Beef Stew (see page 278). If you don't take an afternoon nap, try it. They are a great way to conserve that precious Qi.

Above all, give yourself enough time to eat and digest. Many of my patients also find it helpful to massage the abdominal area before and after a meal, a proven way to get the Qi flowing.

If your digestive disturbances persist, an individualized herbal prescription from your Chinese practitioner may be necessary.

PHYSICAL EXERCISE FOR THE SENIOR PHASE OF LIFE

Even though your body may grow older, it's important to keep moving. Too much stagnation and too little movement can shrink your muscles and make even simple functions such as walking and lifting a chore.

Three primary organs control your ability to keep muscles toned, bones strong, and joints flexible. First, the Spleen, which is responsible for your muscle tone. Second, the Kidneys, in charge of bone and spinal strength. Finally, the Liver, which gives suppleness to your joints. By protecting these organs you are helping your aging body to support an active lifestyle. This goes for everything from an energetic game of tennis to a few laps in the pool.

A wonderful remedy for aging Liver and Kidney power centers is a medicinal tonic called He Shou Wu Chih. Used for centuries as a natural antiaging treatment, He Shou Wu Chih strengthens tendons, nourishes the Blood, helps with blurred vision, and can also restore hair color.

Starting the day with my internal organ exercises (see page 62) is another great way for seniors to get their Liver, Kidney, and Spleen Qi flowing. Not only do these exercises strengthen all five power centers, they also help to keep muscles and joints flexible and strong. Try following up this simple regimen with a brisk walk for a mile or two to give your Lungs a boost.

It's a routine I practice consistently every day, rain or shine. Because of it, I still maintain the energy I need to meet the demands of a busy life.

BOOSTING MEMORY: THE HEALTHY HEART

Most seniors have had a dreaded "senior moment" at one time or another—that awkward occasion when they can't recall a close friend's name, or their last address. It's an inevitable sign of aging, a hint that their physical body isn't the only thing getting older.

Chinese medicine has a practical explanation for mental lapses, and it begins with the Heart. This is the primary power center in charge of memory and mental acuity. It also houses the Shen, your spiritual armor. Unlike Western medical theory, which associates memory functions with the brain, the Chinese feel it is the Heart and Shen that control mental, emotional, and spiritual functions. This is why you need a strong Heart to stay mentally sharp.

To a lesser extent, the Kidneys also support memory. The Jing contained in this power center helps to control brain development, but, as with other organs, the Kidney function declines as you age.

This means less fuel in the form of Jing and, consequently, the occasional memory lapse.

When the Kidneys and Heart (and Shen) are healthy, your Qi and Blood can pump evenly. Your brain works at optimal efficiency, keeping your thoughts balanced and logical, and your reactions quick and timely.

Let the Heart and Kidneys decline to a Deficient state, however, and your Qi and Blood become weak and stagnant. That opens the door to mental lapses and memory problems that will only grow worse with age.

THE TELLTALE HEART

Science has recently recognized the Heart's connection to memory. In his book *The Heart's Code*, Paul Pearsall, PhD, discovered that heart-transplant recipients actually experience the memories of their organ's donor. This coincides with Chinese theory that says the Heart holds a person's thoughts and memories.

Luckily, there are a number of ways to balance and counteract these declines, and again, it begins with the Heart. To stay strong you need to feed your king, the Heart, with the things you truly enjoy. I always advise my older patients to find an activity that makes them happy. Doing something you love not only strengthens the Heart, it helps keep your brain mentally balanced. Find an organization, a charity, even a part-time job. If you have a skill or special experience you can offer, get going! By helping others, you are stimulating the power of your own mind.

Many seniors want to take that extra step and make a more active contribution to their body-emotion connection. The following is a simple technique, developed by the Institute of Heart Math, that can be very effective.

THE HEART LOCK-IN TECHNIQUE

The Heart Lock-In Technique is designed to increase the Heart's power while rebalancing emotions. It stems from the idea that if you can focus specifically on the Heart, your feelings will be composed and steady.

By practicing this technique for five minutes or more twice a day, you help recharge your emotional system and accumulate energy. It also cushions the impact of daily stress and anxiety. Find a nice quiet place to sit down, and try these three easy steps:

1. Focus your attention on the area of your Heart, and breathe slowly and deeply.
2. Activate and sustain a genuine feeling of appreciation or care for someone or something in your life.
3. Send these feelings of care toward yourself and others. *This energetically benefits them and especially helps to recharge and balance your own system.* If you can, try to maintain this sense of peace and calm for approximately five minutes.

The senior years are a wonderful time to enjoy, especially when you maintain and preserve your personal energy bank account. If you have managed your Qi wisely by making regular deposits into your account and letting it grow, you can stay active and healthy well into your nineties.

Good Health Creates a Lifetime of Opportunity

Nearly every day of his adult life Jim gets up at 4:00 a.m. to make coffee and buy sweet rolls for his staff. He then drives to work at the plumbing company he owns, where he joins his crew on the same regular nine-to-five service calls—never losing his infectious wide-eyed, smile. He rarely gets sick or loses a day of work, yet he still finds time to help out his favorite charities. He even sets aside a generous retirement fund for his secretary and staff.

At eighty years old, Jim is an inspiration to all.

I once asked him how he managed to keep his mind, body, and spirit so well balanced. "It's simple," he said with a laugh. "I love what I do. I love to help people fix their problems."

Jim is an outstanding example of someone who's found his purpose in life. He's at peace with himself and the world around him. There is an age-old Jewish blessing that encapsulates this wisdom perfectly:

If you love yourself and those around you,
You will find perfect health.
If you are happy and healthy,
You will be at peace.
If you are at peace,
You'll find your purpose and success.
Once successful,
Luck and prosperity will come to you.

It's a wonderful example of what everyone should strive for. By doing the things you love you create a harmonious balance that keeps your body healthy no matter where you are in the natural cycle of life.

Attracting the Life You Want

After my patients are in treatment for a while and we work through some of their physical issues, inevitably the conversation moves on to other areas in their life.

It usually comes with a sheepish drop of their head. "I shouldn't be telling you this," they'll say. "It's not at all connected to my health." Then they'll admit that life hasn't been what they had hoped it would be. They talk of missed opportunities, of a longing to do something more fulfilling. The conversation often comes around to the same conclusion: that it's too late to make a change.

"On the contrary," I assure them. "In fact, these kinds of feelings are actually a turning point in Chinese medical treatment. They mean that your awareness, your consciousness, your Shen, is opening up."

When someone is physically and mentally overtaxed, it's difficult to build a career, attract the ideal mate, or make any of the long-term decisions that are necessary in life. Attaining important goals is impossible if overall energy is slow and sluggish. Refill the body's bank account, however, and it's much easier to turn this condition around and move beyond the physical discomfort to see things from a greater perspective.

It happened to me after my own cancer surgery. After my physical issues cleared, I finally had the energy and mental clarity to take a long, hard look at myself. My life's purpose became clear and within a few short years, I was able to make some big changes: I moved to the United States, set up house, and started my own practice. At the age of forty-five my life opened up and things virtually fell into place.

How can you reach this place of clarity and ease, and access the bigger picture?

Chinese medicine talks of an ancient pattern that maximizes this stage in the healing process: a synergy between three of our most important treasures: Jing, Qi, and Shen.

Maximizing Your Jing, Qi, and Shen

Let's say you are suffering an energy blockage. Nothing is moving; you have a veritable traffic jam in the midst of your power centers.

The process of receiving nutrients has been cut off, and now your emotions are caught in a repetitive cycle. With a blockage like this, no wonder the future seems cloudy.

Without energy, your body-kingdom is like a flickering lightbulb. Lacking full power, it strains to fulfill its purpose. Jing, Qi, and Shen are the power sources your system needs to operate at its full potential. This is why Chinese medicine regards them as the "Three Treasures." They form the spiritual and physical foundation of human life, and are ultimately responsible for how you think and feel.

- **Jing** is your liquid foundation, or life *essence*, and includes all of your genetic and reproductive information.
- **Qi** is your electricity, your life *force*, and moves throughout your body by means of Blood and the meridians.
- **Shen** is your wisdom, consciousness, and awareness; your life *spirit*; it is centered primarily in your Heart and brain.

Shen dwells in the upper half of the body, whereas Jing is created and stored in the lower half. Qi is the connective force that unites them into a powerful system.

Each of these treasures depends on the other two. If there isn't enough Jing, or if your Qi is Deficient, there won't be enough energy to "pump" Blood to the brain. This often leads to unbalanced or disturbed thinking.

If you are having difficulty with life's bigger decisions, it could mean your Jing, Qi, and Shen are not operating cohesively, and thereby not circulating to the organs that need them. Under these circumstances you may lose purpose and give up on the things you once felt were so important. It's a recipe for frustration and regret that only leads to more bad choices.

To keep this from happening, you need to make sure the energy pathways are open and that Qi and Blood can circulate freely. An open Shen leads to increased creativity and intuition and keen intuition. You'll feel calmer and able to see the big picture, and those important life decisions will be much easier to make. Only when your Jing, Qi, and Shen are operating in harmony can the body, mind, and soul be fully engaged and will you be at peace.

Remember that no matter what life phase you are in, every person has the capacity to change. When you commit to loving your body, that is the moment when you begin attracting the life you want.

Finding Your Purpose

Every person wants and needs a true purpose in life.

Remember my friend Jim? At eighty he is an example of someone who has found his purpose. He is content, compassionate, and helps others. His body, mind, and spirit are active and he still does what he loves. In China we would say his Jing, Qi, and Shen balanced in ideal harmony.

To unlock your own purpose, the key is right there in these inherited gifts. Treat your Qi, Jing, and Shen well, and you will discover a wealth of energy and wisdom.

Crossing the Bridge: Laura

When Laura came to see me she was single, a talented artist, juggling a high-pressure job in print advertising for a major movie studio. She was suffering from chronic cystitis as well as exhaustion and painful menstrual symptoms.

Laura was at the top of her field, making a great income, yet she was depressed and constantly sick. A tough boss and tight deadlines made her feel as though she was constantly "plugging holes in the dam." Her social life was in shambles; though single, she didn't even have time to date.

Laura confessed to me that her job killed her spirit. Deep down, Laura wanted to be an independent artist again, yet the thought of starting over, and struggling to make ends meet, was not appealing. She couldn't see beyond her fatigue and the vicious work cycle that trapped her.

I asked her to be patient. "I'll help you build a bridge to the reality you want, but you need the strength to get to the other side," I said.

First, Laura needed to work on her body, and the rest would eventually come. We started with her Kidneys, restoring her digestion to create more Blood and Qi. In that way her Shen could open up and let her wisdom blossom.

Sure enough, about a year later, Laura crossed her "bridge," leaving her job and going on to become an accomplished artist. In the process, she met her husband and soul mate, and now lives a simpler but far more rewarding life.

LIKE YOUR JOB

If you think you hate your job it may be because you are Deficient and lacking energy to carry it out. Before you make an important decision, such as leaving your position, balance your body-kingdom. You'll find that everything seems much clearer and your job future brighter.

If you're having trouble deciding what direction to take, the best strategy is to stay calm, and begin to strengthen your body. Start with some simple meridian exercises, a visual meditation, perhaps some dietary changes, and then reassess. If your physical and emotional issues seem insurmountable, see a Chinese practitioner. His or her knowledge and experience can open the door to a fulfilling life and lasting health.

Celebrate Your Life

If there's one last piece of advice I can give, it is this: *Live in the here and now.*

Very often my patients confess they wish they could go back in time, back to when their body was younger, more resilient, and full of energy. But then I ask them, "Where is the joy in reliving a past you've already lived?" To make life's journey long and rewarding, one has to follow nature's road map and honor each phase of growth along the way.

Aging doesn't mean that you have to stop doing the things you love. It just means you need to listen to your body and fully live in the moment. Each day is another opportunity to tune in to your unique capabilities, to be intimately aware of the internal life force shared by every living thing.

Your vital life force, or Qi, is the most precious thing you own. It's important to celebrate this gift and keep it safe from outside invaders. Follow nature's rhythms, eat well, exercise, and stay centered, and your Qi will remain vibrant and strong.

Of course everyone experiences periods of weakness and vulnerability. If you decide that you need help, a Chinese practitioner is there to find the source of your imbalance, and reconnect you to the natural energy flow within.

Traditional Chinese medicine works. It's not better than Western medicine, nor is it inferior. It is a close cousin living side by side with the latest medical discoveries and modern techniques. It is a three-thousand-year-old healing art that will help you release the emotions and energies that are keeping you blocked. At its best it not only reverses illness but connects your mind, body, and spirit as one.

After a lifetime of healing many thousands of people, I have written this book, which represents my hope—that you will take all that you've learned here and bring it into your daily life. I want you to understand the emotional source of your physical symptoms. I want you to be aware of your imbalances and catch a problem before it becomes a costly medical crisis. I want you to love your body and have the confidence and power you need to accomplish anything. But most of all, I want you to have total and lasting health.

DR. TING'S TOTAL HEALTH ESSENTIALS

FOUR PHASES OF LIFE

- **Infancy through Childhood:** A time of *growth* and *flux* in the power centers
  - **Eating habits:** Eat small portions with an emphasis on protein, and drink four cups of water a day
  - **Immune system:** Protect your power centers from extreme temperature.
  - **Mental state/nerves:** Do not overstimulate.
  - **Environment:** Spend thirty minutes a day in nature.
- **Puberty through Adolescence**: A time of vigorous growth, with an emphasis on *building strength* and *stamina*
  - **Emotions:** Release anger and frustration.
  - **Diet:** Eat three meals, and limit Heating foods such sugar and alcohol.
  - **Exercise:** Stay active, but know your limits. Do not overexercise.
  - **Sex:** Abstain until after high school, stay educated and informed.
- **Young Adult through Middle Age:** Your most active years, a time to manage your energy reserves
  - **Men:** Listen to your body. Get help when you need it.

- **Women:** Most gynecological issues are related to Blood Stagnation, Deficiency, poor diet, and stress.
- **Middle through Senior Years**: The final phase, a time to protect and preserve your vital essences
  - **Diet:** Restore your childhood practices: smaller, digestible meals.
  - **Exercise:** Stay active: do internal organ exercises and low-impact sports.
  - **Heart and Mind:** The Heart should stay healthy to improve memory. Stay socially active and involved.

STRONG JING, QI, AND SHEN = GOOD HEALTH AND A PROSPEROUS LIFE

- **Jing** is your liquid foundation, or life *essence,* and it includes all of your genetic and reproductive information.
- **Qi** is your electricity, your life *force,* and it moves throughout your body by means of Blood and meridians.
- **Shen** is your life *spirit,* your wisdom, consciousness, and awareness; it resides in your upper body, particularly the Heart and brain

Appendix 1: How to Find a Chinese Practitioner

When looking for a Chinese practitioner, it's important that he or she is licensed and properly certified. In general, training programs in the United States differ from school to school, and can range from three to four years. The title issued to the doctor varies by state is most often *licensed acupuncturist* (L.Ac.), but may be *registered acupuncturist* (R.Ac.) or *Certified Acupuncturist* (C.A.). Some states offer a combination of the above. If your practitioner also dispenses herbs, please note that each state has differing licensing requirements for this treatment as well. Since laws and regulatory practices vary from state to state, this list of resources may be helpful when seeking a licensed practitioner in your area:

American Association of Acupuncture and Oriental Medicine (AAAOM)

http://www.aaaomonline.org
433 Front Street
Catasauqua, PA 18032
Tel: 1-610-266-1433

The AAAOM provides a listing of qualified practitioners in your area, as well as information on requirements for licensing and practice on a state-by-state basis.

311

National Certification Commission for Acupuncture and Oriental Medicine (NCCAOM)

http://www.nccaom.org
1010 Wayne Avenue, Suite 1270
Silver Springs, MD 20910
Tel: 1-301-608-9680

The NCCAOM will provide you with a list of board-certified practitioners in your area.

The Accreditation Commission for Acupuncture and Oriental Medicine (ACAOM)

http://www.acaom.org
7501 Greenway Center Drive, Suite 760
Greenbelt, MD 20770
Tel: 1-301-313-0855

The ACAOM supplies a list of accredited acupuncture schools that prepare students for the state licensing exams.

Web Sites

htttp://www.acufinder.com

An online acupuncture referral service listing acupuncturists, schools and events.

http://www.acupuncture.com

This site features a comprehensive listing of acupuncture laws and regulations on a state-by-state basis.

Appendix 2: Acupressure Points

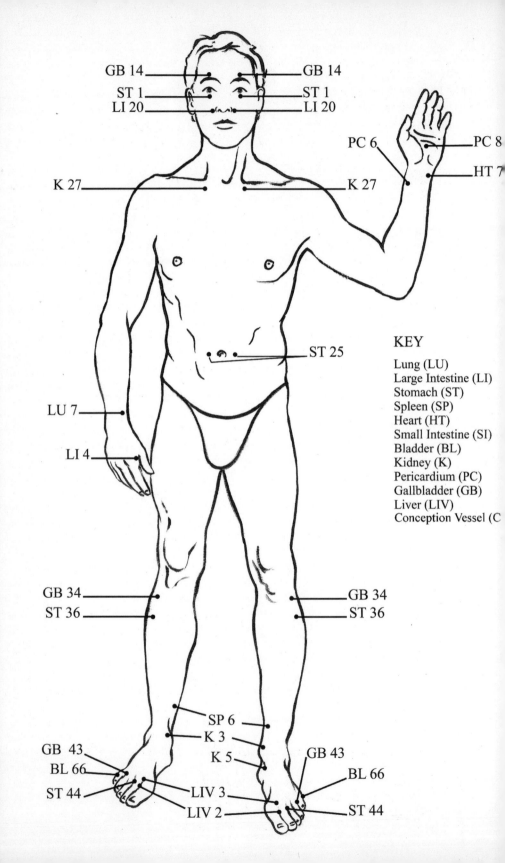

GB 14 — — GB 14
ST 1 — — ST 1
LI 20 — — LI 20

PC 6 — PC 8
— HT 7

K 27 — — K 27

ST 25

LU 7

LI 4

KEY

Lung (LU)
Large Intestine (LI)
Stomach (ST)
Spleen (SP)
Heart (HT)
Small Intestine (SI)
Bladder (BL)
Kidney (K)
Pericardium (PC)
Gallbladder (GB)
Liver (LIV)
Conception Vessel (C

GB 34 — — GB 34
ST 36 — — ST 36

SP 6
K 3
K 5
GB 43 — GB 43
BL 66 — BL 66
ST 44 —
LIV 3 — ST 44
LIV 2 —

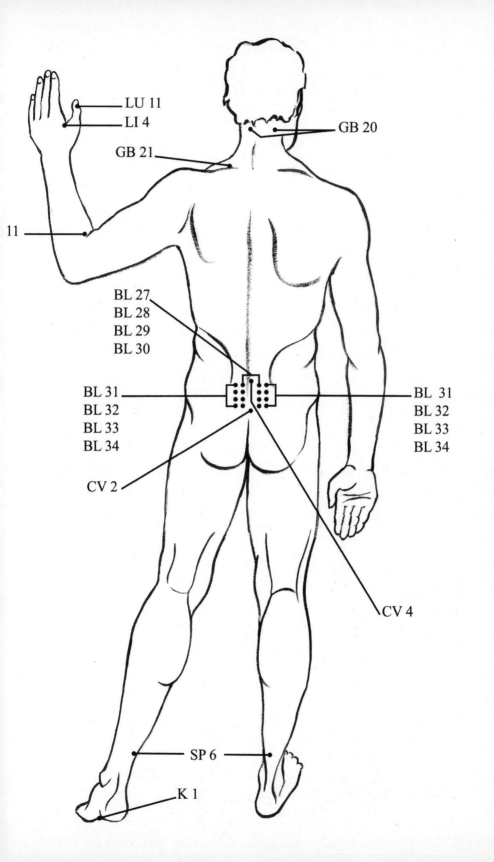

LU 11
LI 4
GB 20
GB 21
11
BL 27
BL 28
BL 29
BL 30
BL 31
BL 32
BL 33
BL 34
BL 31
BL 32
BL 33
BL 34
CV 2
CV 4
SP 6
K 1

Glossary

Acupoint Specific access point or energy gateway on the body through which energy flows.

Acupressure Chinese healing method designed to rebalance or unblock the flow of energy along meridians within the body. Manual pressure is applied at specific points to redirect the flow along these meridians.

Acupuncture Chinese healing method designed to rebalance or unblock the flow of energy within the body. Acupuncture needles are placed into the body to activate, manipulate, and free the energy, or Qi.

Blood The Chinese concept of Blood is that of a dense, nutritious substance formed by food and oxygen and fundamental to all facets of physical and mental health. It is the material form, or mother, of Qi.

Cold (Coldness) One of the Five Temperature Devils. A decrease in body temperature accompanied by cold extremities, poor circulation, and pale skin.

Channels Invisible pathways along which Qi travels, supplying energy and nourishment to the organs and various systems throughout the body. (Also called meridians.)

Damp (Dampness) One of the Five Temperature Devils. A moist condition that affects the body with such symptoms as sluggishness and tired, heavy limbs.

Deficient (Deficiency) A lack of Blood, Qi, or Fluids within the body, causing inadequate function of the organs.

Dry (Dryness) One of the Five Temperature Devils. Symptoms include dehydration, extreme thirst, and dry skin and hair.

Excessive (Excess) Too much of something, either Yin, Yang, Heat, Cold, or Fluids.

External Used to describe an illness that manifests itself on the outside of the body, such as colds, flu, fevers, or skin eruptions.

317

Internal Used to describe an illness that manifests itself on the inside of the body. These ailments affect the Qi and Blood, as well as Internal and External Organs.

Fire Excess Heat, usually associated with the Liver, Stomach, or Heart.

Five Emotions Five primary emotions are considered the major cause of illness: anger, sadness, worry, fear, and joy.

Fluids All the secretions in the body *except* Blood, such as saliva, sweat, tears, spinal fluids, and mucus.

Heat (Hot) One of the Five Temperature Devils. An increase in body temperature; symptoms can include fever, constipation, skin eruptions, and hypertension.

Jing The vital essence responsible for reproduction, development, and growth.

Meridians Energy channels or meridians that run along the body. There are seven primary channels along the front of the body, and seven along the back.

Moxa Dried mugwort.

Moxibustion Mugwort is burned and applied in the form of a cigarlike tube, and when lit it gives off a smoky, musky odor. To disburse it over a larger area, it is burned in a box that is placed on the body.

Organs Twelve major organs in the body: Liver, Heart, Spleen, Lungs, Kidneys, Small Intestine, Large Intestine, Urinary Bladder, Stomach, Gall Bladder, and Triple Heater.

Phlegm A mucus-like substance created when the body fluids are not in harmony with one another.

Qi The Chinese term for the universal life force that is present throughout the body and runs along its energy meridians.

Qigong A series of moving and static exercises designed to open up the flow of Qi.

Shen One's internal spirit and one of the Three Treasures of Chinese medicine. Encompasses enthusiasm for life, charisma, behavior, and coherent speech as well as vitality and joy.

Stagnation Congestion of Qi, Blood, or Fluids due to Cold, Heat, or food.

Stomach Fire Excess Heat within the Stomach.

Tan A thick glue of undigested food or other waste that transforms into the building blocks for body fat.

TCM Abbreviation for "traditional Chinese medicine."

Three Treasures The three energy components—Jing, Qi, and Shen—that make up one's spiritual and physical self.

Wei Qi Defensive guard that protects the body from outside viruses and pathogens.

Wind One of the Five Temperature Devils. Similar to nature's wind, a dry condition with symptoms that can include heat and nervousness.

Yang One of two opposites in Chinese philosophy, indicating an active, moving, warming energy. (See *Yin*.)

Yin One of two opposites in Chinese philosophy, indicating a passive, reflective, and cooler energy. (See *Yang*.)

Zhang-Fu The Chinese term used to collectively describe the twelve organs of the body.

Further Reading

Animal Acupuncture

Schwartz, Cheryl. *Four Paws Five Directions*. Berkeley: Celestial Arts, 1996.

Chinese Food Therapy

Flaws, Bob. *Curing Hay Fever Naturally with Chinese Medicine*. Boulder, CO: Blue Poppy Press, 1997.

Leggett, Daverick. *Helping Ourselves: A Guide to Traditional Chinese Food Energetics*. Totnes, UK: Meridian Press, 1995.

Lu, Henry. *Chinese System of Food Cures*. New York: Sterling Publishing House, 1986.

Pitchford, Paul. *Healing with Whole Foods: Asian Traditions and Modern Nutrition*. Berkeley: North Atlantic Books, 2002.

Yeh, Pearl, and Timothy Yeh. *Seasonal Food Medicine*. Upland, CA: Yeh's Center of Natural Medicine Inc., 1996.

Chinese Massage

Pritchard, Sarah. *Chinese Massage Manual*. New York: Sterling Publishing, Inc., 1999.

Chinese Medicine

Beinfeld, Harriet, and Efrem Korngold. *Between Heaven and Earth: A Guide to Chinese Medicine*. New York: Ballantine, 1992.

321

Dougans, Inge. *The New Reflexology.* New York: Marlowe and Company, 2006.

Elias, Jason, and Katherine Ketcham. *Chinese Medicine for Maximum Immunity.* New York: Three Rivers Press, 1998.

Kaptchuk, Ted. *The Web That Has No Weaver.* Chicago: Contemporary Books, 2000.

Lu, Nan. *A Woman's Guide to a Trouble-Free Menopause.* New York: HarperCollins, 2000.

————. *A Woman's Guide to Healing from Breast Cancer.* New York: Avon Books, 1999.

McNamara, Sheila. *Traditional Chinese Medicine.* New York: Basic Books, 1996.

Ni, Maoshing. *The Yellow Emperor's Classic of Medicine.* Boston: Shambala, 1995.

Ody, Penelope. *Practical Chinese Medicine.* New York: Sterling Publishing Inc., 2000.

Scheid, Volker. *Currents of Tradition in Chinese Medicine 1626–2006.* Seattle: Eastland Press, Inc., 2007.

Williams, Tom. *The Complete Illustrated Guide to Chinese Medicine.* Boston: Element, 1996.

Chinese Sexual Therapy

Gach, Michael Reed. *Acupressure for Lovers.* New York: Bantam Books, 1997.

Chinese Patent Medicine

Taylor, Mark. *Chinese Patent Medicines.* Santa Cruz: Global Eyes International Press, 1998.

Chinese Psychology

Hammer, Leon. *Dragon Rises, Redbird Flies.* Barrytown, New York: Station Hill Press, 1990.

Hicks, Angela, and John, Hicks. *Healing Your Emotions.* London: Thorsons, 1999.

Emotional Freedom Technique (EFT)

Feinstein, David, Donna Eden, and Gary Craig. *The Promise of Energy Psychology.* New York: Tarcher, 2005.

Look, Carol. *Attracting Abundance with EFT: Emotional Freedom Techniques.* Bloomington, IN: Author House, 2005.

Mercola, Joseph, and Ron Ball. *Freedom at Your Fingertips: Get Rapid Physical and Emotional Relief with the Breakthrough System of Tapping.* Fredericksburg, VA: Inroads Publishing, 2008.

Energy Medicine

Boryshenko, Joan. and Miroslav Boryshenko. *The Power of the Mind to Heal,* Carlsbad, CA: Hay House, Inc., 1994.

Eden, Donna. *Energy Medicine.* New York: Penguin Putnam, Inc., 1998.

Hay, Louise. *Heal Your Body: The Mental Causes for Physical Illness and the Metaphysical Way to Overcome Them.* Carlsbad, CA: Hay House Inc., 1984.

Pert, Candace. *Molecules of Emotion: The Science Behind Mind-Body Medicine.* New York: Scribner, 1997.

Feng Shui

Mainini, Simona. *Fengshui for Architecture.* Philidelphia, PA: Xlibris Corporation, 2004.

Too, Lillian. *Lillian Too's Easy to Use Feng Shui: 168 Ways to Success.* Salt Lake City: Sterling, Inc., 1999

Flower Essences

Hasnas, Rachelle. *Pocket Guide to Bach Flower Essences.* Freedom, CA: The Crossing Press, 1997.

Kaminski, Patricia, and Richard Katz. *Flower Essence Repertory.* Nevada City, CA: The Flower Essence Society, Inc., 2004.

Herbs, Herbology

Tierra, Leslie. *Healing with the Herbs of Life.* Berkeley: Crossing Press, 2003.

Useful Addresses and Web Sites

Herbal Companies

BRION HERBS CORPORATION
9200 Jeronimo Road
Irvine, CA 92618
1-800-333-4372
1-949-587-1238
http://www.brionherbs.com

HEALTH CONCERNS
8001 Capwell Drive
Oakland, CA 94621
1-800-233-9355
1-510-639-0280

KAN HERB COMPANY
6001 Butler Lane
Scotts Valley, CA 95066
1-831-438-9450
http://www.kanherbs.com

KPC HERBS
16 Goddard
Irvine, CA 92618
1-949-727-4000
1-800-KPC-8199
http://www.kpc.com

PLUM FLOWER BRAND
Mayway Corporation
1338 Mandela Parkway
1-510-208-3113
Oakland, CA 94607

PLANET HERBS
P.O. Box 275
Ben Lomond, CA 95005
1-800-717-5010
http://www.planetherbs.com

SEVEN FORESTS
2017 SE Hawthorne Boulevard
Portland, OR 97214
1-503-233-4907
http://www.itmonline.org

Flower Essences

FES FLOWER ESSENTIALS
P.O. Box 1769
Nevada City, CA 95959
1-800-548-0075
Fax: 1-530-265-6467

Lifestyle Tools

COLOR THERAPY
Jean Ann Allen
Acupressure, Sound, and Color Specialist
337 South Beverly Drive, Suite 111
Beverly Hills, CA 90212
1-310-552-9543

EMOTIONAL FREEDOM TECHNIQUE
http://www.emofree.com
http://www.eftexpert.com
http://www.patriciacarrington.com
http://www.caroltuttle.com
http://www.carollook.com

VISUALIZATION TECHNIQUES
http://www.creatavision.com
http://www.heartmath.org

FENG SHUI
American Feng Shui Institute
111 N. Atlantic Boulevard, Suite 352
Monterey Park, CA 91754
fsinfo@amfengshui.com

http://www.Lillian-too.com
http://www.fastfengshui.com
http://www.about-fengshui.com
http://www.professional-house-clearing.com

QIGONG
The International Chi Kung/Chi Gong Directory
P.O. Box 19708
Boulder, CO 80308
1-303-442-3131

Traditional Chinese Medicine National Organizations for Diseases or Ailments

ADDICTION
National Acupuncture Detoxification Association
1-888-765-6232 (1-888-765-NADA)

National Association of Addiction Treatment Providers
313 W. Liberty Street, Suite 129
Lancaster, PA 17603
1-717-392-8480
Fax: 1-717-392-8481
E-mail: rhunsicker@naatp.org

TEEN SEX EDUCATION
Sexuality Information and Education Council of the United States
http://www.siecus.org

BREAST CANCER
Traditional Chinese Medicine World Foundation
396 Broadway
Suite 501
New York, NY 10013
1-212-274-1079

Acknowledgments

We owe an enormous debt of gratitude to the many generations of Ting family doctors who provided the foundation and knowledge that helped Esther on her path. She is honored to follow in their footsteps and continue their vital work.

Special thanks to Esther's great-grandfather, Dr. Ding Ganren, who founded China's first teaching hospital and college of traditional Chinese medicine, and who inspired her to understand the human body. To her grandfather, Dr. Ding Zhongying, who gave Esther her spiritual foundation and taught her to forgive and forget. To her father, Dr. Ding Ji Hua, who encouraged her to love all patients, and to Esther's mother, Dr. Ying Yu Wen, who gave her the gifts of tolerance, consistency, and faith.

Our sincere gratitude also to all of the teachers and mentors who passed down their vast knowledge of Chinese medical wisdom: Dr. Yai Shou Cheng, who empowered his students to bring Chinese medicine to the world; Dr. Zhang Ying, who encouraged Esther to study hard and master the healing herbs; Dr. Timothy Yeh, who helped to further her studies in the United States; and to Dr. Yan De Xin and Dr. Cai Xiao Sun, who kept Esther up to date with the latest research.

Without the superhuman efforts of Larry Gay this book would not be. He has masterfully shaped, formed, and guided the manuscript from beginning to end. Thank you.

Our appreciation to Dr. Barbara Solomon, for introducing us to each other some ten years ago, and to Debbie Gruber for urging us to teach the class that became the groundwork for this book. Thanks also to Mary Foote and Nancy Lamb for their treasured friendship and writing expertise; and to Jacuie Nemor, Dalia Allen-Meeter, and Elizabeth Ralser for their dedicated and untiring editing efforts.

We would also like to thank our editors: Matthew Lore for believing in this project and getting it off the ground, Renee Sedliar for her warm support and expertise in shepharding it through the process, and the entire Da Capo team for their thoughtful and dedicated work. Our tremendous gratitude to our agent Malaga Baldi for her sage advice and insights, and to Barbara Kolo for her superb artwork.

A heartfelt thanks to our families: Esther's son, Peter, and his family; Dr. Denis Ting, Rhoda Ting, and the extended Ting family; to Marianne's parents, Frank and Tine Jas; her in-laws, John and Bobbie Gay; the Svensons, the Jases, the Summers, and the Powells. We are forever indebted to you for all your love and support.

Finally, this book would not be possible without the dedicated Chinese philosophers and physicians who have been diligently studying the human body for the last three thousand years.

Index